The Artificial Intelligence in Digital Pathology and Digital Radiology: Where Are We?

The Artificial Intelligence in Digital Pathology and Digital Radiology: Where Are We?

Editor

Daniele Giansanti

MDPI • Basel • Beijing • Wuhan • Barcelona • Belgrade • Manchester • Tokyo • Cluj • Tianjin

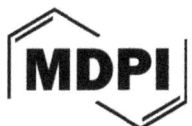

Editor
Daniele Giansanti
Centro nazionale per le
tecnologie innovative in
sanità pubblica
Istituto Superiore di Sanità
Rome
Italy

Editorial Office
MDPI
St. Alban-Anlage 66
4052 Basel, Switzerland

This is a reprint of articles from the Special Issue published online in the open access journal *Healthcare* (ISSN 2227-9032) (available at: www.mdpi.com/journal/healthcare/special_issues/AI_Digital_Pathology_Radiology).

For citation purposes, cite each article independently as indicated on the article page online and as indicated below:

LastName, A.A.; LastName, B.B.; LastName, C.C. Article Title. *Journal Name* **Year**, *Volume Number*, Page Range.

ISBN 978-3-0365-4310-9 (Hbk)
ISBN 978-3-0365-4309-3 (PDF)

© 2022 by the authors. Articles in this book are Open Access and distributed under the Creative Commons Attribution (CC BY) license, which allows users to download, copy and build upon published articles, as long as the author and publisher are properly credited, which ensures maximum dissemination and a wider impact of our publications.

The book as a whole is distributed by MDPI under the terms and conditions of the Creative Commons license CC BY-NC-ND.

Contents

About the Editor . . . . **vii**

Preface to "The Artificial Intelligence in Digital Pathology and Digital Radiology: Where Are We?" . . . . **ix**

Daniele Giansanti
The Artificial Intelligence in Digital Pathology and Digital Radiology: Where Are We?
Reprinted from: *Healthcare* **2020**, *9*, 30, doi:10.3390/healthcare9010030 . . . . **1**

Adrian Gillissen, Tonja Kochanek, Michaela Zupanic and Jan Ehlers
Medical Students' Perceptions towards Digitization and Artificial Intelligence: A Mixed-Methods Study
Reprinted from: *Healthcare* **2022**, *10*, 723, doi:10.3390/healthcare10040723 . . . . **5**

Daniele Giansanti, Ivano Rossi and Lisa Monoscalco
Lessons from the COVID-19 Pandemic on the Use of Artificial Intelligence in Digital Radiology: The Submission of a Survey to Investigate the Opinion of Insiders
Reprinted from: *Healthcare* **2021**, *9*, 331, doi:10.3390/healthcare9030331 . . . . **19**

Daniele Giansanti and Francesco Di Basilio
The Artificial Intelligence in Digital Radiology: Part 1: The Challenges, Acceptance and Consensus
Reprinted from: *Healthcare* **2022**, *10*, 509, doi:10.3390/healthcare10030509 . . . . **33**

Francesco Di Basilio, Gianluca Esposisto, Lisa Monoscalco and Daniele Giansanti
The Artificial Intelligence in Digital Radiology: *Part 2: Towards an Investigation of acceptance and consensus* on the Insiders
Reprinted from: *Healthcare* **2022**, *10*, 153, doi:10.3390/healthcare10010153 . . . . **47**

Maria Rosaria Giovagnoli and Daniele Giansanti
Artificial Intelligence in Digital Pathology: What Is the Future? *Part 1: From the Digital Slide Onwards*
Reprinted from: *Healthcare* **2021**, *9*, 858, doi:10.3390/healthcare9070858 . . . . **63**

Maria Rosaria Giovagnoli, Sara Ciucciarelli, Livia Castrichella and Daniele Giansanti
Artificial Intelligence in Digital Pathology: What Is the Future? *Part 2: An Investigation on the Insiders*
Reprinted from: *Healthcare* **2021**, *9*, 1347, doi:10.3390/healthcare9101347 . . . . **77**

Bhakti Patel and Amgad N. Makaryus
Artificial Intelligence Advances in the World of Cardiovascular Imaging
Reprinted from: *Healthcare* **2022**, *10*, 154, doi:10.3390/healthcare10010154 . . . . **87**

Daniele Giansanti
Comment on Patel, B.; Makaryus, A.N. Artificial Intelligence Advances in the World of Cardiovascular Imaging. *Healthcare* 2022, *10*, 154
Reprinted from: *Healthcare* **2022**, *10*, 727, doi:10.3390/healthcare10040727 . . . . **99**

Bhakti Patel and Amgad N. Makaryus
Reply to Giansanti, D. Comment on "Patel, B.; Makaryus, A.N. Artificial Intelligence Advances in the World of Cardiovascular Imaging. *Healthcare* 2022, *10*, 154"
Reprinted from: *Healthcare* **2022**, *10*, 735, doi:10.3390/healthcare10040735 . . . . **103**

Magbool Alelyani, Sultan Alamri, Mohammed S. Alqahtani, Alamin Musa, Hajar Almater and Nada Alqahtani et al.
Radiology Community Attitude in Saudi Arabia about the Applications of Artificial Intelligence in Radiology
Reprinted from: *Healthcare* **2021**, *9*, 834, doi:10.3390/healthcare9070834 105

Seongmin Kim, Hwajung Lee, Sanghoon Lee, Jae-Yun Song, Jae-Kwan Lee and Nak-Woo Lee
Role of Artificial Intelligence Interpretation of Colposcopic Images in Cervical Cancer Screening
Reprinted from: *Healthcare* **2022**, *10*, 468, doi:10.3390/healthcare10030468 115

Siti Shaliza Mohd Khairi, Mohd Aftar Abu Bakar, Mohd Almie Alias, Sakhinah Abu Bakar, Choong-Yeun Liong and Nurwahyuna Rosli et al.
Deep Learning on Histopathology Images for Breast Cancer Classification: A Bibliometric Analysis
Reprinted from: *Healthcare* **2021**, *10*, 10, doi:10.3390/healthcare10010010 125

About the Editor

Daniele Giansanti

Dr. Giansanti has received: an MD in Electronic Engineering at Sapienza University, 1991, Rome; a PhD in Telecommunications and Microelectronics Engineering at Tor Vergata University, 1997, Rome; the Academic Specialization in Cognitive Psychology and Neural Networks at Sapienza University, Rome, 1997; and his Academic Specialization in Medical Physics at Sapienza University, Rome, 2005. Dr. Giansanti was in charge of the Design of VLSI Asics for DSP in the Civil Field (1991–1997) during his MD and PhD studies, and he served as CAE-CAD-CAM system manager and Design Engineer in the project of electronic systems (Boards and VLSI) for Warfare at Elettronica spa (1992–2000), one of the leaders in this military field. More importantly, he also conducts various research at ISS (the Italian NIH) (2000–today) in the following fields: (1) biomedical engineering and medical physics with the design and construction of wearable and portable devices (three national patents); (2) telemedicine and e-Health: technology assessments and the integration of new systems in the fields of tele-rehabilitation, domiciliary monitoring, digital pathology, and digital radiology; (3) Mhealth: recent interests in the fields of smartphone and tablet technology in health care, with particular focus on the opportunities and relevant problems of risks, abuse, and regulation; (4) acceptance and consensus in the use of robots for assistance and rehabilitation; (5) challenges and acceptance regarding the use of artificial intelligence in digital radiology and digital pathology; (6) cybersecurity in the health domain; and (7) technologies for frail and disabled people. He is a Professor at Sapienza and Catholic University in Rome, where he teaches several courses and is the tutor for several theses. He is a Board Editor and reviewer for several journals. He has 126 indexed publications on Scopus, more than 200 contributions as monographies and chapters, and contributes to congresses.

Preface to "The Artificial Intelligence in Digital Pathology and Digital Radiology: Where Are We?"

As a result of the incredible advances brought about by information and communication technology, as seen today in eHealth and mHealth, many new applications of both organ and cellular diagnostics are now possible. In the era of digitalization, we can focus specifically on the prospects of digital radiology and digital pathology.

Digital radiology includes the use of diagnostic imaging tools for organs based on systems compatible with digital imaging and communications in medicine (DICOM), known as DICOM-compliant. This comprehends not only instruments whose image formation processes are based on fields of interaction that use ionizing radiations, but also instruments based on ultrasound and magnetic fields (nuclear magnetic resonance), for example.

Digital pathology, on the other hand, includes the use of digital processes related to instrumentation for cell diagnostics, which mainly take two forms: histological and cytological. In this case, we refer to digital histology and digital cytology. However, other processes for digitizing information in biomedical laboratories are also included in this area, such as those relating to the integration of cytometric reports.

Artificial intelligence is extending into the world of both digital radiology and digital pathology, and involves many scholars in the areas of biomedicine, technology, and bioethics. These scholars are interested in the potential applications of artificial intelligence in feature recognition, diagnostics, automatic recognition, quality control, and other fields, including the limits and the associated problems. There is a particular need for scholars to focus on innovations in this field and the problems hampering integration in the health domain into a robust and effective process in stable health care models. Many professionals involved in these fields of digital health were encouraged to contribute with their experiences. This book contains contributions from various experts across different fields. Aspects of the integration in the health domain have been addressed. Particular space was dedicated to overviewing the challenges, opportunities, and problems in both radiology and pathology. Clinal deepens are available in cardiology, breast cancer, and colonoscopy. Dedicated studies based on surveys investigated students and insiders, opinions, attitudes, and self-perception on the integration of artificial intelligence in this field. We dedicate this book to all those involved with different roles in radiology and pathology processes in healthcare.

Daniele Giansanti
Editor

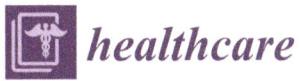 healthcare

Editorial

The Artificial Intelligence in Digital Pathology and Digital Radiology: Where Are We?

Daniele Giansanti

Centre Tisp, Istituto Superiore di Sanità, Via Regina Elena 299, 00161 Roma, Italy; daniele.giansanti@iss.it;
Tel.: +39-06-4990-2701

Citation: Giansanti, D. The Artificial Intelligence in Digital Pathology and Digital Radiology: Where Are We? *Healthcare* 2021, 9, 30. https://doi.org/10.3390/healthcare9010030

Received: 25 December 2020
Accepted: 28 December 2020
Published: 31 December 2020

Publisher's Note: MDPI stays neutral with regard to jurisdictional claims in published maps and institutional affiliations.

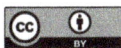

Copyright: © 2020 by the author. Licensee MDPI, Basel, Switzerland. This article is an open access article distributed under the terms and conditions of the Creative Commons Attribution (CC BY) license (https://creativecommons.org/licenses/by/4.0/).

1. The Digital Radiology and Digital Pathology

Thanks to the incredible changes promoted by Information and Communication Technology (ICT) conveyed today by *electronic-health* (*eHealth*) and *mobile-health* (*mHealth*), many new applications of both organ and cellular diagnostics are now possible. Today, in the era of digitalization, we prefer to speak specifically about the prospects of *digital radiology* and *digital pathology*.

The first one includes the use of diagnostic imaging tools for organs and/or body functions based on systems compatible with *Digital Imaging and COmmunications in Medicine* (DICOM), or as it is commonly said, *DICOM-compliant*. In particular, *digital radiology* (DR) includes not only those instruments whose image formation processes are based on the interaction fields that use ionizing radiation, but also instruments of different types such as, for example, those instruments based on ultrasound (ultrasound) or magnetic fields [1,2] (nuclear magnetic resonance).

The second one, *digital pathology* (DP) includes the use of digital processes related to instrumentation for cellular diagnostics, mainly (but not only) in two forms: histological and cytological [3,4]. We can also speak of *digital histology* and *digital cytology* as the two major components of the DP, however, the DP also includes other processes for digitizing information in a biomedical laboratory such as by way of non-exhaustive example such as those relating to the integration of cytometric reports.

2. General Actual Developments of *Digital Radiology*, *Digital Pathology*, and the Artificial Intelligence

Of course, a detailed analysis of the perspectives of the DR and the DP would deserve two separate treatments. However, in light of the objective of this contribution, brief considerations of a fundamental nature are reported. In recent years, the DR has opened up both to new forms of construction and/or reconstruction applications of artificial reality and artificial intelligence (also related).

As far as artificial reality is concerned, we are seeing more and more applications of augmented and/or virtual reality. For example, in [5,6], they are some available ones that use the DICOM file from computed tomography) and/or magnetic resonance imaging to return to the surgeon on support augmented reality viewers during an operation (as for a fighter pilot), for example, the exact placement of blood vessels or a nerve. Virtual reality applications in the so-called virtual colonoscopy or in all those endo-cavitary diagnostic applications, where it is possible to create a real virtual journey (thanks to the processing of *voxels* starting from the file saved in DICOM), are now routine. This possibility of processing *voxels* to create environments of artificial reality also finds wide application today in the two sectors of three-dimensional reconstruction (3D) and simulation and training in surgery. In fact, by processing the *voxels*, it is possible to transform the DICOM file into a file of the standard format for the 3D printing called stereolithography (STL) and to print models of organs and tissues (e.g., bones). For example, it is now routine to print skeletal parts to design replacement bioengineering parts. An example of such applications can be found in the treatment of pelvic fractures caused by osteoporosis or bone cancer: the 3D model of the pelvis is printed and then bioengineering grafts are designed with biomaterials on the same model. As for simulation and training in surgery, it is now possible to use technologies for augmented and virtual reality combined with systems for restoring the perception of force, called force-feedback. Therefore, the system will give a perception of force-feedback associated, for example, with the liver to the surgeon who trains in liver surgery. Furthermore, *Artificial Intelligence* (AI) is bursting into the world of the DR and is affecting many scholars both in the world of technologies and bioethics. These scholars are interested both in the potential of feature recognition, automatic recognition, and quality control, but also in the limitations and related problems and the new applications in the fields described above and the related research activities [7–9]. Surely, the evolutions of digitalization processes in the world of the DP [3,4] are taking place at a slower rate than in the world of DR, especially because the DP has not adapted to the DICOM standard (DICOM WSI in this case) with the same readiness as the DR. However, it has been shown how digitization processes in this area [4–6] can favor the decision processes and the training, which uses a very strong component of *mHealth* in environments where training is based on smartphone viewers to which the image is sent from a centralized digital microscope. Furthermore, artificial reality can certainly be of support by providing tools to navigate around cellular and/or tissue elements. Furthermore, the AI, as discussed for the DR, is breaking into the world of the DP, and also in this case affecting many scholars both in the world of innovative technologies [10] and bioethics.

3. What Future Awaits Us for Artificial Intelligence in Digital Radiology and Digital Pathology?

Recent advances in AI have led to the conclusion that artificial intelligence could be very useful in DR very soon in routine applications [7]. Researchers have developed *deep learning neural networks* that can identify pathologies in radiological images such as bone fractures and potentially cancerous lesions [8,9]. The *deep learning* is advancing rapidly, and is a much better technology than previous approaches to medical imaging, however, the best systems currently live up to human performance and are used only in research environments. Radiological practice would certainly benefit from systems capable of rapidly reading and interpreting multiple images because the number of images has increased much faster in the last decade than the number of radiologists. It is evident that in DR, the amount of work is very high, so every solution able to reduce it could be welcome, decreasing the costs and improving the process. Like other AI systems, systems used in radiology perform individual tasks and are trained and used for specific image recognition tasks. However, thousands of activities are needed to fully identify all potential outcomes in medical images, and only some of these can be performed by the AI today. In addition, image interpretation work includes only a few of the tasks performed by radiologists. They also consult with other doctors for diagnosis and treatment, treat diseases, perform image-guided medical interventions, tailor the exam on the patient's needs, discuss outcomes, activities, and procedures with patients and many other activities. *Therefore, in DR it is important to understand what the role of AI is and the help it can provide us.* Scientists in DP benefit from combining histopathological data obtained, analyzed, and shared with other sources of clinical data such as that obtained from *omics*, *historical clinical data*, and *demographic data*. However, it is difficult to integrate the data collected in different formats that do not combine in a useful way [3,4]. For example, medical records are mostly kept in an unstructured text format. AI is helping to integrate information from these multiple sources [5,6,10]. Natural language processing, a branch of AI, is being used, for example, to extract pertinent details from written notes from the entire slide representation. Methodologies of AI are being developed to help integrate data from all sources, not just imaging. In addition, AI is being used to help decrease the errors that are made in diagnostic pathology. Before the birth of DP, the diagnosis from tissue samples always rested on the competence of medical professionals. AI can try to reduce the error rate in the diagnostic processes.

4. What Are the Aspects to Be Explored and to Deepen?

It is clear that AI, albeit with a different speed, is making a major breakthrough in both DR and DP.

In both sectors:

- *The development involves both the world of imaging diagnostics and the related ones described above.*
- *A large number of image databases and in any case data patterns in general are being developed on which researchers can build and test their models/architectures of AI.*
- *A new direction certainly concerns the fusion of the contemporary approach based on AI on organ and cellular/histological diagnostics and affect both the radiology and biomedical laboratory.*
- *There has been a tremendous research activity and impulse during the Covid-19 pandemic [11].*
- *mHealth is emerging through the use of targeted Apps.*

This incredible development involves many scholars both from the world of technologies and bioethics. These scholars are interested in both the potential in applications of AI in feature recognition, diagnostics, automatic recognition, integration in the new processes including the quality control, but also to the limits and the related problems. It is important to face and contribute to this, which has a broad spectrum ranging from the continuous innovation aspects including the recent ones correlated to the Covid-19 pandemic up to the problem of the last "yard" of the AI, depending on the acceptance of all actors from the health operators up to the patients.

Conflicts of Interest: The authors declare no conflict of interest.

References

1. Giansanti, D. Teleradiology Today: The Quality Concept and the Italian Point of View. *Telemed. J. E. Health* **2017**, *23*, 453–455. [CrossRef]
2. Orlacchio, A.; Romeo, P.; Inserra, M.C.; Grigioni, M.; Giansanti, D. *Guidelines for Quality Assurance and Technical Requirements in Teleradiology; English Translation and Revision of Rapporti ISTISAN 10/44*, Rapporti ISTISAN 13/38; Istituto Superiore di Sanità: Roma, Italy, 2013; pp. 1–33.
3. Giansanti, D. How Image Enhancement Is Allowing New Chances for Digital-Cytology in Telemedicine and e-Health. *Telemed. J. E. Health.* **2017**, *23*, 615–617. [CrossRef] [PubMed]
4. Giansanti, D. *Digital Cytology: An Experience with Image-Enhancement and Tablet Technologies*; Rapporti ISTISAN 16/46; Istituto Superiore di Sanità: Roma, Italy, 2016; pp. 1–32.
5. Giansanti, D. *Diagnostic Imaging and E-Health: Standardization, Experiences and New Opportunities*; Rapporti ISTISAN 17/10; Istituto Superiore di Sanità: Roma, Italy, 2019; pp. 1–60.
6. Giansanti, D. *Diagnostics Imaging and M-Health: Investigations on the Prospects of Integration in Cytological and Organ Diagnostics*; Rapporti ISTISAN 20/1; Istituto Superiore di Sanità: Roma, Italy, 2019; pp. 1–66.
7. Jalal, S.; Nicolaou, S.; Parker, W. Artificial intelligence, radiology, and the way forward. *Can. Assoc. Radiol. J.* **2019**, *70*, 10–12. [CrossRef] [PubMed]
8. Hosny, A.; Parmar, C.; Quackenbush, J.; Schwartz, L.H.; Aerts, H.J.W.L. Artificial intelligence in radiology. *Nat. Rev. Cancer* **2018**, *18*, 500–510. [CrossRef] [PubMed]
9. European Society of Radiology (ESR). What the radiologist should know about artificial intelligence-an ESR white paper. *Insights Imaging* **2019**, *10*, 44. [CrossRef] [PubMed]
10. Jahn, S.W.; Plass, M.; Moinfar, F. Digital Pathology: Advantages, Limitations and Emerging Perspectives. *J. Clin. Med.* **2020**, *9*, 3697. [CrossRef]
11. Senbekov, M.; Saliev, T.; Bukeyeva, Z.; Almabayeva, A.; Zhanaliyeva, M.; Aitenova, N.; Toishibekov, Y.; Fakhradiyev, I. The Recent Progress and Applications of Digital Technologies in Healthcare: A Review. *Int J. Telemed. Appl.* **2020**, *2020*, 8830200. [CrossRef]

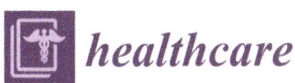 healthcare

Article

Medical Students' Perceptions towards Digitization and Artificial Intelligence: A Mixed-Methods Study

Adrian Gillissen [1,*], Tonja Kochanek [1], Michaela Zupanic [2] and Jan Ehlers [1]

[1] Institute for Didactics and Educational Research in Health Care, Department of Medicine, Faculty of Health, Witten/Herdecke University, 58455 Witten, Germany; tonja.kochan3k@gmail.de (T.K.); jan.ehlers@uni-wh.de (J.E.)
[2] Interprofessional and Collaborative Didactics, Department of Medicine, Faculty of Health, Witten/Herdecke University, 58455 Witten, Germany; michaela.zupanic@uni-wh.de
* Correspondence: adrian.gillissen@uni-wh.de; Tel.: +49-23-02926-78603

Abstract: Digital technologies in health care, including artificial intelligence (AI) and robotics, constantly increase. The aim of this study was to explore attitudes of 2020 medical students' generation towards various aspects of eHealth technologies with the focus on AI using an exploratory sequential mixed-method analysis. Data from semi-structured interviews with 28 students from five medical faculties were used to construct an online survey send to about 80,000 medical students in Germany. Most students expressed positive attitudes towards digital applications in medicine. Students with a problem-based curriculum (PBC) in contrast to those with a science-based curriculum (SBC) and male undergraduate students think that AI solutions result in better diagnosis than those from physicians ($p < 0.001$). Male undergraduate students had the most positive view of AI ($p < 0.002$). Around 38% of the students felt ill-prepared and could not answer AI-related questions because digitization in medicine and AI are not a formal part of the medical curriculum. AI rating regarding the usefulness in diagnostics differed significantly between groups. Higher emphasis in medical curriculum of digital solutions in patient care is postulated.

Keywords: medical students; perceptions; digitization in medicine; artificial intelligence

---

1. Introduction

Digitized health care systems require all players to acquire suitable knowledge of how to use these technologies appropriately and to understand their implications on patient management in general as well as on a case-by-case basis. Medical knowledge is expanding exponentially and requires physicians to be constantly up-to-date and quickly communicate, analyze, and recall medical information from numerous sources. Since 1955, artificial intelligence (AI) has had more and more support from stakeholders in the medical field and elsewhere to generate and investigate digital data at a speed and precision never seen before [1]. Digitization, including AI, changes not only the physician's work but requires also that medical education must align with these quite different health care contexts compared to traditional teaching concepts [2]. Further, non-analytical, humanistic aspects of medicine come under scrutiny and compete with digital technologies. The acceptance of advanced technologies by students and health professionals and the weighing of its usefulness is extremely important once this modality of healthcare delivery became an integral part of mainstream healthcare. Acceptance, keenness to use the digital tools, knowledge and skills, as well as an exuberance to utilize digital tools as an inherent way of service delivery by healthcare professionals, particularly by doctors, help facilitate the integration of eHealth and thus enhance the quality of health care [3]. This means that among other institutions, such as universities, more and more should ensure that all active players, including medical students, acquire knowledge, skills, and attributes to work with these digital tools by an adaptation of curricula of education [4–7]. Although scientific

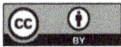

publication on AI has increased since the beginning of this century, integration into medical curriculum for better understanding of AI algorithms and how to maximize their use is rudimentary [8].

Studies have demonstrated the usefulness of AI algorithms in various medical specialties, including radiology, ophthalmology, dermatology, pathology and pulmonary medicine [9,10]. Regardless of the paucity of evidence to support digital tools, including AI, in day-to-day routine in patient care and irrespective of the likeliness of the rapid emergence of numerous AI applications, students' contact with university and medical courses teaching these concepts are rare. Surveys investigating students' attitudes towards field-specific AI are just emerging [9,11–14]. In some studies, students indicate their intention to abstain from medical fields, such as radiology, where AI was regarded as a potential competitor to physicians' work [9,11]. However, most wish for the integration of digital applications and smart algorithms as well as their use in clinical practice and integration into their curriculum [2,8,9,15,16].

No study has tested—to the best of the authors' knowledge—whether students' perceptions regarding various aspects of eHealth (digitization including AI) depends on only their personal beliefs or also on other confounding factors. Lee et al. (2021) found there is little consensus on what and how to teach AI in medical education, requiring further research to facilitate greater implementation of standardized aspects of digital medicine and AI in the medical curriculum [17], while German universities offer medical studies either a science-based focus (SBC, science-based curriculum) or a problem-based curriculum (PBC), which gives the unique opportunity to evaluate students' perceptions in this regard, allowing the analysis of compounding factors not only regarding gender and training stage but also the curriculum type.

2. Aim of the Study

The overall objective of this study was to investigate today's medical students' attitudes towards AI and other digital working tools. We wanted to understand if age, gender, semester level, and curriculum type influence their views. This study also assembled information on students' understanding of AI algorithms and digital applications in health care and assessed their level of confidence in working alongside these tools after graduation into patient care. It is our belief that this information may possess the means to employ digital tools, including AI, into the curriculum of medical students efficiently, enhancing their confidence in using them and therefore better equipping our future physicians with sufficient knowledge.

3. Materials and Methods

3.1. Design

In order to best pursue the aim of this study, an exploratory mixed-method design was used [18,19]. We used a sequential exploratory strategy in which a qualitative study phase was followed by a quantitative survey [20–22]. The intention of the initial qualitative component of the first study phase was to collect information about medical students' perceptions regarding digitization and artificial intelligence (AI) in medicine. This was then integrated into the second study phase consisting of a nationally representative sample of the same sort of cohort. Thus, the first phase informed the next in an additive form, but it is not a parallel design per se. This design is widely used to evaluate the effect of community influence in which one method enriches the other method for comprehensibility [23]. For the first phase, themes were extracted from the literature related to medical students' perceptions regarding digitization in medicine, eHealth, and AI. The following topics were extracted:

- Patient-related themes: digitization in patient self-management and interaction with the health-care system;
- Physician-related themes: communication, information, managing health data, AI and machine learning, and patient and administrative management;

- Student-related themes: course of digitization and AI in medical school and attitudes towards the digitization of medicine.

This information was then analyzed in two discussion group sessions among all authors, and a resulting interview guide with a set of open questions about medical students' perceptions of digitization and artificial intelligence was constructed. This set consisted of three main themes, and the authors agreed on adjunct questions for each theme to probe explanations of the answers more deeply. The list was piloted with five medical students, allowing further refinement prior to the interviews. The items are listed in Table S1.

For the second, quantitative study phase, this findings were used to develop an internet-based survey to confirm the results of the qualitative part quantitatively but not to generate a formal theory [21,24]. Every item that was mentioned in more than two interviews was translated into a question. All questions were reviewed by the authors separately for content validity. This is seen as an objective judgment about the construct of an instrument, ensuring the instrument's relevance to the study's aim and elucidating how to express phrases, the wording of questions, and understanding the researcher's intended concept [25,26]. The items were then tested through a pilot study consisting of a group of 4 pre- and 4 clinical students, mediated by the authors to understand how they perceive the subject of interest and in order to finalize the list of items. The comments and suggestions were integrated, and overlaps were avoided, resulting in the final construct of questions.

3.2. Participants and Selection Criteria in Each Phase

In Germany, digitization and AI are not a formal part of the medical curriculum although some medical students may have acquired relevant information about these themes during courses with patient presentation (hidden curriculum). All in all, medical students were, in terms of the curriculum, digitally naive. All participants of the first phase were students from their 1st to 6th year (undergraduate, 1st to 2nd year; graduate, 3rd to 6th year) from German universities. The inclusion criteria were their active study of medicine and their agreement for their voluntarily participation. In the same way, the exclusion criteria were suspension their studies as well as other exceptional situations. Prior to start, informed consent was obtained, which was followed by the collection of telephone numbers and email addresses. Convenience sampling was used. They were selected purposely and consecutively, in part by snowball until theoretical saturation was reached. All were approached personally by the authors. Once started, no interviewee dropped out of the interview, which lasted about 30 min. Semester number and interview time were comparable between the two groups. Table 1 summarizes the baseline characteristics of all participants. All quotations in this paper are translations from German language into English.

For the second, quantitative study phase, identical inclusion/exclusion criteria applied. The online survey was sent to all medical faculties in Germany, from which most forwarded the survey invitation by email to about 80,000 medical students to fulfill the principle of maximum diversity through convenience sampling method. Each contained an invitation letter and an information sheet. To avoid a potentially low response rate, 280 Amazon vouchers, each for EUR 25 per completed survey, were offered as incentives, which were distributed by way of a lottery. The samples of qualitative and quantitative studies are comparable in age and percent number of PBC/SBC students but slightly different in gender distribution and frequency of undergraduate or graduate semester (Table 1).

3.3. Analytical Strategy of the Qualitative Phase

The interviews consisted of semi-structured face-to-face or telephone interviews. They took place between November 2019 and March 2020 at the Witten/Herdecke University. Students replies were transcribed as verbatim texts and analyzed using an inductive coding approach according to Mayring's principles, as also exploited by others [27–29], aided by the use of Quirkos 2.4 software (Quirkos, Edinburgh, United Kingdom www.quirkos.com

accessed on 11 August 2021). A thematic analysis was performed by all authors and themes linked and grouped to develop a schema for interpreting the data, ensuring rigor in analysis [30]. When the perceptive content of the interviewees replicated itself, data saturation was assumed, and the interview series was terminated. A.G. and J.E. read each transcript up to three times to familiarize themselves with the contents and in order to analyze the content properly. Data were then independently coded (Table 2). The process involved the recognition of patterns and connections across the data and the establishment of themes and sub themes that were pertinent and applicable to the whole data set. Differences were discussed under the facilitation of TK until general consensus was achieved. Reflexivity was maintained by the three researchers involved in the data analysis, being cognizant throughout of their own personal context as, respectively, practicing clinicians and educators and of any potential effect this may have had on their interpretation of the data. Using this methodological approach, the authors followed a quantitative inquiry approach, which is also the cornerstone of grounded theory [31].

Table 1. Characteristics of the study cohorts.

Parameter	Specifics (Qualitative Study)	Specifics (Quantitative Study)
Students	$n = 28$	$n = 1053$
Age (years)	24.76 ± 3.05	23.7 ± 3.9
Gender distribution	♀ $n = 17$ (60.7%)	♀ $n = 779$ (74.0%)
	♂ $n = 11$ (36.3%)	♂ $n = 274$ (26.0%)
Semester		
(1–4) = Undergraduate	$n = 10$	$n = 438$ (41.6%)
(5–12) = Graduate	$n = 18$	$n = 615$ (58.4%)
Interview time (minutes/interviewee)	29.5 ± 2.6	25–30
PBC students	$n = 13$ (46.4%)	$n = 490$ (46.5%)
Gender	♀ $n = 5$ (38.5%), ♂ $n = 8$ (61.5%)	♂ $n = 153$ (31.2%), ♀ $n = 337$ (68.8%)
Age	26.9 ± 4.1	23.8 ± 4.0
SBC students	$n = 15$ (53.6%)	$n = 563$ (53.5%)
Gender	♀ = 12 (80.0%), ♂ = 3 (20.0%)	♂ = 121 (21.5%), ♀ = 442 (78.5%)
Age	22.60 ± 2.03	23.7 ± 3.8

3.4. Analytical Strategy of the Quantitative Phase

The questionnaire consists of a total of 71 questions in eight sections: (A) sociodemographics, (B) preliminary activity, (C) admission to medical studies, (D) medical studies, (E) expectations of studies/profession, (F) learning, (G) future and digitization, and (H) patient and error management. Likert scale questions (ranging from 0 = decline/do not know to 7 = completely agree), questions with a percent scale from 0–100, and questions with the option of three answers (do not know, false, fully agree) were used. An item was considered a "firm perception" when the mean response was within one-third of the lowest/highest possible answer scores. The survey took place between September 2020 and January 2021.

3.5. Statistics

Statistical analysis was performed in the quantitative study part using SPSS (V27). Descriptive statistics are presented in percentages. An unpaired, two-tailed Wilcoxon rank-sum test was carried out to compare the responses relating to perceptions in digitization in medicine and AI. Group comparators were curriculum type (PBC vs. SBC), gender (female vs. male), and semester levels. A p-value of less than 0.05 was considered statistically significant.

Table 2. Codes used in the qualitative study part.

Code	Descriptors	Subthemes
Health Apps	Professional health apps for medical decision finding. Lay health apps giving diagnostic advise and therapeutic control	Doctor's competitor, Doctor's assistant Technical challenges Erroneousness (misleading) Patient's assistant Information tool Patient–doctor alienation Economization of consultations
Wearables	Electronic devices to track physical metrics, consumer wearables	Effects on self-determination Medical device Motivation tool Self-controlling Health consciences Monitoring tool for physical fitness
Telemedicine	Telecommunication technology for remote health care	Simplification of doctor–patient interaction Monitoring tool 24/7 surveillance Amelioration of patient quality of life Enhances patient's independence
Digitization in patient management	Electronic software solutions to aid the health care	Peer-to-peer communication Patient management Patient records Literature search Data management and transfer Digital literacy of users
Data protection	Safeguarding of important information	Data misuse Transparent patient Unnecessary restrain Patient health card
Robotics in medicine	Use of computerized or automated devices in health care	Doctor's assistant Doctor's competitor Support in diagnostic and analytic procedures Alienation of patients Legal responsibility
AI	Computer- or software-driven machines to perform activities normally thought to require intelligence	Doctor's assistant Doctor's competitor Support in diagnostic and analytic procedures Legal responsibility Distrust Lack of information

4. Results

Students estimated that digital health cannot and will never replace traditional health services and medical consultations in total, but it will change the way doctors and patients will deal with each other.

> "I think, in the digital age the personal contact is particularly important. Many [patients] can easily search for information in the Internet using their mobile or smartphone. But it is something different when patients and doctors interact with each other and communicate in person. The physician can do a physical examination, take care of the patient directly which allows also emphatic interaction into the patient's psyche".

This perception is mirrored by the data from the quantitative study. Digitization in general is not seen as a competition for doctors but as an accessory tool to improve their performance, save time, and make their work easier. Male students are somewhat more skeptical than women (Table 3). Male students see AI more as an encumbrance than as useful assistance.

Table 3. Response (sum ± STD) from Likert scale responses to given questions. Statistical group comparison using the unpaired, two-tailed Wilcoxon rank-sum test.

Questions	PBC (n = 490)	SBC (n = 563)	Male (n = 274)	Female (n = 779)	Undergraduate (n = 438)	Graduate (n = 615)
Digitization makes doctors in diagnostic workup dispensable. 0 = do not know, 1 = false, 7 fully agreed.	2.50 ± 0.91	2.60 ± 1.00	2.72 ± 1.09	2.49 ± 0,91	2.54 ± 0.990	2.56 ± 0.94
group comparison	p = 0.096		p = 0.007 (alpha = 0.003)		p = 0.588	
Medical decisions can be digitally supported but must be finalized through the doctors because only they can fully assess the outcome. 0 = do not know, 1 = false, 7 fully agreed.	5.99 ± 1.29	5.91 ± 1.32	5.95 ± 1.43	6.00 ± 1.26	5.92 ± 1.45	6.02 ± 1.96
group comparison	p = 0.971		p = 0.940		p = 0.925	
Health apps and computer algorithms are for patients disturbing (0) or coherent (100).	50.1 ± 22.6	47.5 ± 22.4	51.4 ± 24.7	47.7 ± 21.6	45.4 ± 22.5	51.1 ± 22.2
Group comparison	p = 0.066		p = 0.018 (*)		p < 0.0001	
Health apps/computer algorithms are in medicine debilitating (0) or supportive (100).	63.4 ± 18.9	60.5 ± 18.6	66.0 ± 20.4	60.4 ± 17.9	60.9 ± 19.3	62.62 ± 18.33
group comparison	p = 0.003		p < 0.001		p = 0.325	
Digital self-diagnostics are for patients deleterious (0) or useful (100).	38.1 ± 23.4	35.2 ± 20.8	38.0 ± 22.5	36.0 ± 21.9	33.2 ± 21.7	39.0 ± 22.0
group comparison	p = 0.105		p = 0.244		p < 0.0001	
The multiplicity of health apps cause confusion. 0 = do not know, 1 = false, 7 fully agreed.	3.88 ± 1.96	4.25 ± 2.04	4.17 ± 1.96	4.02 ± 2.03	3.96 ± 2.02	4.16 ± 2.00
	p = 0.001		p = 0.449		p = 0.083	
Wearables can replace 24 h ECG and others in medical diagnostics. 0 = do not know, 1 = false, 7 fully agreed.	2.74 ± 1.35	2.70 ± 1.30	2.84 ± 1.29	2.68 ± 1.29	2.75 ± 1.39	2.70 ± 1,28
Group comparison	p = 0.540		p = 0.114		p = 0.753	

* = non-significant after Bonverroni correction of alpha error.

Although the semi-structured interview was based only on three major topics, students discussed six related sub-themes in lengths and with great enthusiasm, which were categorized as the digital patient, digitization in doctor–patient interaction, technical aspects of digitization, robotics in medicine, artificial intelligence (AI), and digitization in university.

4.1. The Digital Patient

Students show a well-balanced attitude or are even enthusiastic regarding the advantages of internet-using patients (or "ePatients", as Masters, 2017, put it [32]). Concerns are related to potentially unreliable and non-certified internet sources eventually causing confusion in the patient–doctor relationship, particularly when the doctor disagrees with the patient's internet inquiry (Figure S1). In general, they believe that informed patients can more easily be integrated into the doctor's decision making.

> "That means that the patient visits the doctor well informed. Informed patients gave thoughts to their symptoms, in a positive but also possibly in a negative sense. As a matter of principle I like informed patients as long as patients are open for further suggestions and towards the doctor's medical advice. On the flip side can such lay information interfere with doctor's intention because it cause a behavioral bias on the patient side towards certain diagnostic procedures and therapies".

Some doubt the reliability of health apps and the practical usefulness for doctors, particularly those who lack the necessary willingness and technical understanding.

> "But I must say, for example just for me, I am not very technically avid and only partially trained or have only meager digital skills".

Students emphasize that apps might be used as a useful information source for doctors as well as for patients although they question the accuracy of mobile health applications for patients [33], and they caution a possible fallout for the utilization on the health care system (Table S2). Only a minority of the students knew that common activity trackers are not certified medical devices, precluding them from being used as such. Students argue in favor of the use of those devices, mainly citing the stimulating effect on a physical activity and their perception of these devices as a positive motivation tool for healthy lifestyle (Table S3).

Although the quantitative study part did not find ample differences, SBC students tend to have slightly more restrictive attitude than PBC students towards patients' use of consumer health apps. They seem, although by and large having a more positive than a timid attitude, more reluctant regarding the use of medical apps to aid diagnosis and therapy by doctors. Interestingly, the perception for or against the use of digital applications in medicine for patients and doctors seems to change. While undergraduate students have more critical and restrained perceptions, graduate students see more of the positive side most likely due to their comparably higher training level. Thus, group differences of perceptions were mainly driven by semester rank rather than by gender or by educational type (Table 3).

4.2. Digitization in Doctor–Patient Interaction

In interviews, participants verbalized indifferent knowledge of telemedicine inventions. Positive aspects included the simplification of doctor consultations, particularly in sparsely populated areas, possible 24/7 doctor access, and the medical on-the-spot support of paramedics (Table S3, supplement). They doubted that electronic communication services would enhance the doctor–patient relationship because direct and physical doctor–patient interaction will always be the cornerstone of patient care. However, increasing electronic communications, in contrast to face-to-face contact between patients and the doctor but also between stakeholders in medicine, is seen as unavoidable in modern days. The computer screen might be on the verge of becoming more essential than the physical presences of the patient, or personal interactions might weaken, such as the deterioration of experience of physical examination and medical history taking due to the dominance of electronic data and the loss of individual patient characteristics.

Students of the quantitative study part had positive attitudes toward telemedicine, with women having the most favorable views. Digital communication and attentiveness toward patients despite working with a computer and electronic networking were seen neither overly optimistically nor pessimistically within all groups (Table 4). Interestingly, all of them think that digital solutions in patient care might ease doctor–nurse communications but not personal doctor–patient interactions. Male students favor high-tech medicine themes in the curriculum, while female students prefer the personal patient–doctor-interaction and use their senses in physical examinations rather than relying on impersonal technical tools for the diagnostic workup (Figure 1). All students, and particularly those at the graduate level, express their willingness to improve healthcare, including its digital solution concepts.

Table 4. Response (sum ± STD) from Likert scale responses to given questions. Statistical group comparison using the unpaired, two-tailed Wilcoxon rank-sum test.

Questions	PBC (n = 490)	SBC (n = 563)	Male (n = 274)	Female (n = 779)	Undergraduate (n = 438)	Graduate (n = 615)
Digital networks (including telemedicine) make face-to-face medical consultations unnecessary. 0 = do not know, 1 = false, 7 = fully agree.	2.40 ± 0.86	2.41 ± 0.84	2.57 ± 1.05	2.35 ± 0.76	2.43 ± 0.92	2.39 ± 0.80
Group comparison	$p = 0.567$		$p = 0.006$ (alpha = 0.003)		$p = 0.925$	
Would it be problematic for you as a doctor that you work more at the computer instead of directly interacting with the patient? 1 = yes, 2 = no, 3 = do not know.	1.42 ± 0.73	1.41 ± 0.74	1.36 ± 0.70	1.44 ± 0.75	1.41 ± 0.74	1.42 ± 0.74
Group comparison	$p = 0.692$		$p = 0.116$		$p = 0.641$	
What do you think: Does digitization in medicine reduce (0) or enhance (100) personal doctor–doctor communication?	49.8 ± 26.2	49.2 ± 25.7	52.1 ± 27.4	48.6 ± 25.3	48.8 ± 25.8	50.0 ± 26.0
Group comparison	$p = 0.705$		$p = 0.076$		$p = 0.496$	
What do you think: Do digital networks increase (0) or decrease (100) doctor–nurse communication?	40.5 ± 22.3	36.7 ± 20.7	40.3 ± 22.5	37.8 ± 21.2	37.5 ± 21.3	39.2 ± 21.8
Group comparison	$p = 0.010$ *		$p = 0.213$		$p = 0.170$	
How do you deal with a non-perfect health care system: Do you try learn the pitfalls in order to adapt yourself (0), or do you try to improve an imperfect system actively (100)?	58.8 ± 24.6	57.4 ± 23.9	55.1 ± 26.2	59.1 ± 23.5	60.6 ± 23.6	56.2 ± 24.5
Group comparison	$p = 0.316$		$p = 0.068$		$p = 0.003$	
Digitization in medicine lacks confidentiality and breaches private data security. 0 = do not know, 1 = false, 7 = fully agree.	3.08 ± 1.20	3.17 ± 1.26	3.07 ± 1.17	3.15 ± 1.25	3.22 ± 1.29	3.07 ± 1.18
Group comparison	$p = 0.296$		$p = 0.155$		$p = 0.025$ *	
Do you regard the statutory health card susceptible for fraud (0) or a tool to improve quality of patient-centered care (100)?	67.8 ± 20.1	66.7 ± 20.7	69.5 ± 21.1	66.4 ± 20.1	65.6 ± 19.9	68.4 ± 20.8
Group comparison	$p = 0.467$		$p = 0.011$ *		$p = 0.007$ *	

* = non-significant after Bonverroni correction of alpha error.

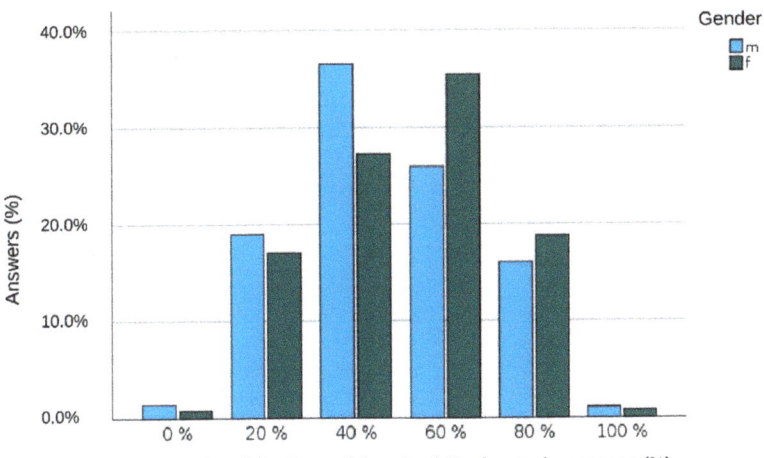

Figure 1. Male (m) students favor high-tech medical themes in the curriculum more than women do (f).

4.3. Technical Aspects of Digitization

Students had a balanced attitude towards technical and operational aspects of digitization in patient care, citing critical but also positive aspects as summarized in Table S5. All students were aware of privacy issues and considered informed consent as essential. However, they do not appear to give privacy issues a high ranking order because both groups cite that many people easily give away personal information voluntarily, such as in social media or while using open Internet access gates (Table S6). They even consider privacy regulations as somewhat cumbersome for the doctors to whom patients have to give private information anyway.

> "I don't know why data protection concerns in medicine are so widely discussed. Well, I don't care if my health insurance and physicians can see my diseases because they get this information anyway. I you ask me ... I tell my physician my medical problems anyway which is a courtesy making life easier".

Most students reject the notion that digitization interferes substantially with privacy. They further regard data storage on personal health insurance cards as more helpful for doctors' work and as offering less vulnerability for abuses. They see a high potential for enhancing medical quality, which out-weighs the risks. Students in earlier semesters view cybersecurity and women in particular view insurance cards with more concern than do graduate students or men, respectively (Table 4).

4.4. Robotics and AI in Medicine

The interviewees did not clearly distinguish robotics and machine learning from other AI applications. Most students draw their knowledge about AI and medical robotic systems either from personal experience or interest by citing the movie *I, Robot*, from casual encounters during courses, or from reports in the general media. Particularly, SPC students expressed critical attitudes against AI and robotic applications in medicine, which they regard as inhuman. In contrast, PBC students saw AI and robotics as supportive, even expressing excitement. Both groups strongly emphasized that AI and robots will never replace doctors and the warm heartedness of human-to-human interaction although AI might be a formidable competitor particularly in radiology, pathology, and other fields were AI has been shown to outperform even specialists (Table S7).

"I think, an intelligent android will never replace a physician because the human element is always the most important component in a doctor-doctor-interaction. Solid social contacts, empathy but also tactfulness is so important which can never be accomplished by a robot".

"I think, that's difficult, because I feel a certain emotional suspiciousness towards technical solutions and AI. But objectively and pragmatically seen, these digital assistance solutions are as a matter of principle a good thing. But emotionally I am quite wary".

"Yes, artificial intelligence is a very fascinating area of cutting edge new technological developments. I think, the we can profit enormously from AI".

Depending on the analyzed group, 10% to almost 40% of students felt uninformed about AI and therefore could not answer the questions of the quantitative survey (Table 5A–C). More PBC than SBC students and more graduate than undergraduate students (non-significant after Bonverroni correction) believe that physicians will lose their medical skills through AI applications. Around 70% of students think that to some extent, AI generates better diagnoses in rare diseases. This study found significant differences between groups: SBC students, women, and undergraduate students are less convinced that AI is superior to physicians (comparison between all groups $p < 0.001$, Table 5B). In contrast to the qualitative part, PBC and SBC students were equally uneasy to disapprove AI (Table 5C). Men as well as undergraduate students had a significant more pessimistic perception towards AI than their counterparts ($p = 0.002$ and $p < 0.002$, respectively).

Table 5. (A–C) Response (% in numeric columns) to given questions. Statistical group comparison using the unpaired, two-tailed Wilcoxon rank-sum test (statistical calculation excluding column 1).

A

Comparator groups	Artificial Intelligence (AI) Leads to Loss of Medical Skills. AI is "Addictive". 1 = Do Not Know, Range of Agreement: 2 = Rejection, up to 7 = Fully Agreement.								
	1	2	3	4	5	6	7	Mean ± STD	p
PBC	13.3	16.7	22.4	16.1	20.0	8.2	3.3	3.50 ± 1.63	$p = 0.033$ * (alpha = 0.016)
SBC	9.9	18.5	21.1	16.2	16.5	23.5	4.3	3.68 ± 1.69	
male	8.8	16.4	23.4	17.2	19.7	11.3	3.3	3.70 ± 1.59	$p = 0.226$
female	12.5	18.1	21.2	15.8	17.6	10.9	4.0	3.57 ± 1.69	
undergraduate	13.9	18.9	21.5	13.9	18.7	9.4	3.7	3.47 ± 1.69	$p = 0.033$ *
graduate	9.8	16.7	22.0	17.7	17.7	12.2	3.9	3.69 ± 1.64	

B

Comparator groups	Particularly in diagnosing orphan diseases, AI outmatches physicians. 1 = Do Not Know, 2 = Range of Agreement: 2 = Rejection, up to 7 = Fully Agreement.								
	1	2	3	4	5	6	7	Mean ± STD	p
PBC	31.8	10.2	15.7	12.0	14.3	12.2	3.7	3.18 ± 1.93	$p < 0.0001$
SBC	32.7	13.7	13.5	12.6	16.3	8.3	2.8	3.03 ± 1.85	
male	28.1	8.4	11.3	12.4	17.9	15.0	6.9	3.56 ± 2.05	$p < 0.0001$
female	33.8	13.4	15.7	12.3	14.5	8.5	1.9	2.94 ± 1.81	
undergraduate	38.4	14.6	12.8	12.8	11.2	7.3	3.0	2.78 ± 1.83	$p < 0.0001$
graduate	28.0	10.2	15.8	12.0	18.4	12.2	3.4	3.33 ± 1.90	

Table 5. Cont.

C	AI will cause disaster rather than being useful. 1 = Do Not Know, Range of Agreement: 2 = Rejection, up to 7 = Full Agreement.								
Comparator groups	1	2	3	4	5	6	7	Mean ± STD	p
PBC	19.0	25.9	30.6	14.5	5.3	3.5	1.2	2.77 ± 1.35	p = 0.158
SBC	17.8	26.1	25.4	17.2	7.5	4.1	2.0	2.91 ± 1.46	
male	6.6	38.0	29.6	12.0	7.7	3.6	2.6	2.97 ± 1.35	p = 0.002
female	22.5	21.8	27.2	17.3	6.0	3.9	1.3	2.79 ± 1.43	
undergraduate	21.5	21.2	24.4	17.4	8.4	4.3	2.7	2.94 ± 1.55	p < 0.001
graduate	16.1	29.4	30.2	15.0	5.0	3.4	0.8	2.88 ± 1.30	

* = non-significant after Bonverroni correction of alpha error.

5. Discussion

This study, based on an exploratory sequential analysis consisting of two study parts, investigated students' attitudes towards various aspects of digitization in medicine with the focus of AI. Germany and many other countries, there is a lack of AI and other digital solutions for patient care in the curriculum, which provides only a cursory reference to AI at the most despite its advantages and its more frequent use [32,34]. Therefore, this study adds to our understanding of what medical students think about chances and challenges of digital tools in patient management as well as the role and future of AI in medicine. Without a structured curriculum, it is difficult to select a solid knowledge base on these themes, which easily can explain the helplessness of some students of our online survey. However, medicine still has to deal with the adoption of digital working tools, including the integration of high-tech simulation into medical curriculum [2,35,36].

The students of the qualitative phase revealed that they drew their knowledge and attitude regarding AI and robotics/machine learning, which they could not clearly differentiate from media and films, and not from courses in the university. Regardless, the qualitative interviews revealed a great array of detailed opinions ranging from AI as a potential competitor in certain medical fields such as radiology, pathology, and others to being supportive for physician's work, liability, and data security. The quantitative study part further revealed for the first time, to the authors knowledge, that students' attitudes are not to be contemplated from a standpoint of structural unity but that distinctive stances exist. Significantly more PBC than SBC and more graduate than undergraduate students think that AI will hamper medical skills of physicians, and significantly more PBC students, male students, and graduate students are convinced of the superiority of AI in detecting rare diseases. Although up 38% of our students could not answer the AI questions in the quantitative survey—initially brought up in the interviews of the qualitative study part—it seems encouraging in comparison to an earlier survey, which reported that about 70% of respondents were unaware of AI topics in medicine [16]. Students of this study expressed a great interest in integrate digitization, AI, and machine learning into the medical curriculum, which is in concordance with earlier reports [9,14–16]. At least the qualitative part of this study matches nicely, from the students' perspective, the attitudes from faculty members in German medical faculties because both postulate an intensification of AI competence in medical training [37].

Healthcare is currently undergoing a digital transformation. Therefore, it is imperative to leverage digital technologies to further improve our understanding of disease pathogenesis, diagnosis, and therapy. Stakeholders in medicine need to believe that new technologies provide an advantage to traditional working structures and are effortless to apply before they will accept them [38,39]. Naturally, people fear that AI may replace clinicians or take their jobs. This attitude might even guide students in their career choice [40,41]. Although this study found differences between groups where undergraduate male and SBC students were significantly more pessimistic, the overall score was quite neutral. Education and training in AI might further contribute to a differentiated view of the pros and cons of these technologies, including smart algorithms in medical applications [42].

This study, nevertheless, has some limitations. This study was conducted at a single institution although students from almost all medical faculties of German universities contributed to this investigation. Self-selection bias may exist due to voluntarily participation. Further, the quantitative survey consisted of about three-fourths women but only one-fourth men, indicating a gender bias corresponding to the gender distributions of students that reflects the situation in many medical faculties. The focus on the German educational system and the fact that only a small fraction of the total number of medical students filled out the online survey makes a generalization of the answers difficult. However, the thorough literature research, the extraction of relevant themes, and the number of interviews performed in the qualitative study phase were comparable to similar qualitative studies, including the number of items included in the survey, which was also accomplished with a similar level of substantiation [43]. The statements of the qualitative study part and questions of the quantitative study part may not always reflect clarity and comprehension. The reason is that those were entirely based on self-reported and subjective measures and therefore did not necessarily follow scientific semantics. The questionnaire for the quantitative study did not undergo a validated validation process. Instead, it underwent a face-validity process by the authors and was pretested in a pilot study, which has been used in other mixed-methods studies [18,36,43].

6. Conclusions

This study represents an important insight regarding digitization and AI-naive students and their perceptions, anxiety, and notions, which were solely based on personal interest, the participation of voluntary courses, or acquired from hidden curriculum. While the attitudes towards digitization in medicine were well-balanced between curricula groups, gender, and training stage, perceptions regarding AI were not. Although in comparison to other studies, AI illiteracy was lower, still, up to almost 40% of participants could not answer AI-related questions although differences in subgroups exist.

7. Implications

There is a broad understanding in the student cohort on the need to integrate education and training in digital applications and AI technologies in medicine. Therefore, it is recommended to integrate themes such as "digitization in medicine" as well as "AI" in the medical curriculum due to their increasing importance in health care. To cope with this aspect, the University Hospital Charité in Berlin started a project called "AI-Campus", which offers courses on a voluntary basis and can be used by every member of medical faculty in Germany. Based on the results of our study, a more formal integration of AI and eHealth themes into health education would not only fit today's requirements of cutting-edge patient care but would also suit medical students' interests, as our study confirmed, and might reduce students' digital illiteracy, which, however, has to be elucidated in another study.

Supplementary Materials: The following supporting information can be downloaded at: https://www.mdpi.com/article/10.3390/healthcare10040723/s1, Figure S1: Students' perceptions on "the internet-affine patient"; Table S1: Interview themes in 28 students of five German universities (qualitative study part); Table S2: Students' perceptions on health apps (lay and professional health apps); Table S3: Students' perceptions on wearables use by patients; Table S4: Students' perceptions on telemedicine; Table S5: Students' perceptions on digitization in patient management (hospital, ambulatory); Table S6: Students' perceptions regarding data security; Table S7: Students' perceptions regarding robotic and intelligence (AI) in medicine.

Author Contributions: A.G.: conceptualization, application to the ethics committee, performing most interviews, transcription of all interviews, coding of the qualitative study part, and writing of the manuscript; T.K.: statistical analysis of the quantitative study part, development and implementation of the online survey and management, revision of the data and the manuscript, and literature research; M.Z.: data interpretation of the online survey, revision of the data and the manuscript, and corrections of the manuscript; J.E.: performing some interviews, analysis of the transcriptions including the coding of qualitative study part, finalization of the manuscript including all final revisions, checking for plagiarism, and supervision. All authors have read and agreed to the published version of the manuscript.

Funding: This research was in part funded by Kreiskliniken Reutlingen GmbH, Germany, grant number UW/H 11.540.

Institutional Review Board Statement: Ethical approval of the study was obtained prior to the first interview from the University Faculty of Medicine and Dentistry Committee for Ethics at the University Witten-Herdecke (# 137/2919). The study was conducted in accordance with the Declaration of Helsinki.

Informed Consent Statement: Informed consent—either written or verbal—was obtained from all subjects involved in the study. All participants of the qualitative study part agreed to the audio recording either verbally or in written form. Confidentiality was warranted through an anonymization process.

Conflicts of Interest: The authors declare no conflict of interest.

References

1. Tran, B.X.; Vu, G.T.; Ha, G.H.; Vuong, Q.-H.; Ho, M.-T.; Vuong, T.-T.; La, V.-P.; Ho, M.-T.; Nghiem, K.-C.P.; Nguyen, H.L.T.; et al. Global Evolution of Research in Artificial Intelligence in Health and Medicine: A Bibliometric Study. *J. Clin. Med.* **2019**, *8*, 360. [CrossRef] [PubMed]
2. Han, E.-R.; Yeo, S.; Kim, M.-J.; Lee, Y.-H.; Park, K.-H.; Roh, H. Medical Education Trends for Future Physicians in the Era of Advanced Technology and Artificial Intelligence: An Integrative Review. *BMC Med. Educ.* **2019**, *19*, 460. [CrossRef] [PubMed]
3. Granja, C.; Janssen, W.; Johansen, M.A. Factors Determining the Success and Failure of EHealth Interventions: Systematic Review of the Literature. *J. Med. Internet Res.* **2018**, *20*, e10235. [CrossRef]
4. Kyaw, B.M.; Posadzki, P.; Paddock, S.; Car, J.; Campbell, J.; Tudor Car, L. Effectiveness of Digital Education on Communication Skills Among Medical Students: Systematic Review and Meta-Analysis by the Digital Health Education Collaboration. *J. Med. Internet Res.* **2019**, *21*, e12967. [CrossRef] [PubMed]
5. Stellefson, M.; Hanik, B.; Chaney, B.; Chaney, D.; Tennant, B.; Chavarria, E.A. EHealth Literacy among College Students: A Systematic Review with Implications for EHealth Education. *J. Med. Internet Res.* **2011**, *13*, e102. [CrossRef]
6. Wentink, M.M.; Siemonsma, P.C.; van Bodegom-Vos, L.; de Kloet, A.J.; Verhoef, J.; Vlieland, T.P.M.V.; Meesters, J.J.L. Teachers' and Students' Perceptions on Barriers and Facilitators for EHealth Education in the Curriculum of Functional Exercise and Physical Therapy: A Focus Groups Study. *BMC Med. Educ.* **2019**, *19*, 343. [CrossRef]
7. Tsukahara, S.; Yamaguchi, S.; Igarashi, F.; Uruma, R.; Ikuina, N.; Iwakura, K.; Koizumi, K.; Sato, Y. Association of EHealth Literacy With Lifestyle Behaviors in University Students: Questionnaire-Based Cross-Sectional Study. *J. Med. Internet Res.* **2020**, *22*, e18155. [CrossRef]
8. Chan, K.S.; Zary, N. Applications and Challenges of Implementing Artificial Intelligence in Medical Education: Integrative Review. *JMIR Med. Educ.* **2019**, *5*, e13930. [CrossRef]
9. Sit, C.; Srinivasan, R.; Amlani, A.; Muthuswamy, K.; Azam, A.; Monzon, L.; Poon, D.S. Attitudes and Perceptions of UK Medical Students towards Artificial Intelligence and Radiology: A Multicentre Survey. *Insights Imaging* **2020**, *11*, 14. [CrossRef]
10. Kaplan, A.; Cao, H.; FitzGerald, J.M.; Iannotti, N.; Yang, E.; Kocks, J.W.H.; Kostikas, K.; Price, D.; Reddel, H.K.; Tsiligianni, I.; et al. Artificial Intelligence/Machine Learning in Respiratory Medicine and Potential Role in Asthma and COPD Diagnosis. *J. Allergy Clin. Immunol. Pract.* **2021**, *9*, 2255–2261. [CrossRef]
11. Gong, B.; Nugent, J.P.; Guest, W.; Parker, W.; Chang, P.J.; Khosa, F.; Nicolaou, S. Influence of Artificial Intelligence on Canadian Medical Students' Preference for Radiology Specialty: ANational Survey Study. *Acad. Radiol.* **2019**, *26*, 566–577. [CrossRef] [PubMed]
12. Cho, S.I.; Han, B.; Hur, K.; Mun, J.-H. Perceptions and Attitudes of Medical Students Regarding Artificial Intelligence in Dermatology. *J. Eur. Acad. Dermatol. Venereol.* **2021**, *35*, e72–e73. [CrossRef] [PubMed]
13. Park, C.J.; Yi, P.H.; Siegel, E.L. Medical Student Perspectives on the Impact of Artificial Intelligence on the Practice of Medicine. *Curr. Probl. Diagn. Radiol.* **2021**, *50*, 614–619. [CrossRef] [PubMed]
14. Oh, S.; Kim, J.H.; Choi, S.-W.; Lee, H.J.; Hong, J.; Kwon, S.H. Physician Confidence in Artificial Intelligence: An Online Mobile Survey. *J. Med. Internet Res.* **2019**, *21*, e12422. [CrossRef] [PubMed]

15. Pinto Dos Santos, D.; Giese, D.; Brodehl, S.; Chon, S.H.; Staab, W.; Kleinert, R.; Maintz, D.; Baeßler, B. Medical Students' Attitude towards Artificial Intelligence: A Multicentre Survey. *Eur. Radiol.* **2019**, *29*, 1640–1646. [CrossRef]
16. Wood, E.A.; Ange, B.L.; Miller, D.D. Are We Ready to Integrate Artificial Intelligence Literacy into Medical School Curriculum: Students and Faculty Survey. *J. Med. Educ. Curric. Dev.* **2021**, *8*, 23821205211024080. [CrossRef]
17. Lee, J.; Wu, A.S.; Li, D.; Kulasegaram, K.M. Artificial Intelligence in Undergraduate Medical Education: A Scoping Review. *Acad. Med. J. Assoc. Am. Med. Coll.* **2021**, *96*, S62–S70. [CrossRef]
18. Curry, L.A.; Krumholz, H.M.; O'Cathain, A.; Plano Clark, V.L.; Cherlin, E.; Bradley, E.H. Mixed Methods in Biomedical and Health Services Research. *Circ. Cardiovasc. Qual. Outcomes* **2013**, *6*, 119–123. [CrossRef]
19. Fetters, M.D.; Curry, L.A.; Creswell, J.W. Achieving Integration in Mixed Methods Designs-Principles and Practices. *Health Serv. Res.* **2013**, *48*, 2134–2156. [CrossRef]
20. Onwuegbuzie, A.J.; Bustamante, R.M.; Nelson, J.A. Mixed Research as a Tool for Developing Quantitative Instruments. *J. Mix. Methods Res.* **2010**, *4*, 56–78. [CrossRef]
21. Pluye, P.; Hong, Q.N. Combining the Power of Stories and the Power of Numbers: Mixed Methods Research and Mixed Studies Reviews. *Annu. Rev. Public Health* **2014**, *35*, 29–45. [CrossRef] [PubMed]
22. Onwuegbuzie, A.J.; Slate, J.R.; Leech, N.L.; Collins, K.M. Conducting Mixed Analyses: A General Typology. *Int. J. Mult. Res. Approaches* **2007**, *1*, 4–17. [CrossRef]
23. Johnson, R.B.; Onwuegbuzie, A. Mixed Methods Research: A Research Paradigm Whose Time Has Come. *Educ. Res.* **2004**, *33*, 14–26. [CrossRef]
24. Warfa, A.-R.M. Mixed-Methods Design in Biology Education Research: Approach and Uses. *CBE Life Sci. Educ.* **2016**, *15*, rm5. [CrossRef] [PubMed]
25. Drost, E. Validity and Reliability in Social Science Research. *Educ. Res. Perspect.* **2011**, *38*, 105–124.
26. Yazdi-Feyzabadi, V.; Nakhaee, N.; Mehrolhassani, M.H.; Naghavi, S.; Homaie Rad, E. Development and Validation of a Questionnaire to Determine Medical Orders Non-Adherence: A Sequential Exploratory Mixed-Method Study. *BMC Health Serv. Res.* **2021**, *21*, 136. [CrossRef] [PubMed]
27. Mayring, P. Qualitative Inhaltsanalyse. In *Handbuch Qualitative Forschung in der Psychologie: Band 2: Designs und Verfahren*; Mey, G., Mruck, K., Eds.; Springer Fachmedien: Wiesbaden, Germany, 2020; pp. 495–511. [CrossRef]
28. Rahm, A.-K.; Töllner, M.; Hubert, M.O.; Klein, K.; Wehling, C.; Sauer, T.; Hennemann, H.M.; Hein, S.; Kender, Z.; Günther, J.; et al. Effects of Realistic E-Learning Cases on Students' Learning Motivation during COVID-19. *PLoS ONE* **2021**, *16*, e0249425. [CrossRef]
29. Tenny, S.; Brannan, G.D.; Brannan, J.M.; Sharts-Hopko, N.C. Qualitative Study. In *StatPearls*; StatPearls Publishing: Treasure Island, FL, USA, 2021.
30. Ryan, G.W.; Bernard, H.R. Data Management and Analysis Methods. In *Handbook of Qualitative Research*; Sage Publications Ltd.: Sauzende Oaks, CA, USA, 2000; pp. 769–802.
31. Tavakol, M.; Torabi, S.; Akbar Zeinaloo, A. Grounded Theory in Medical Education Research. *Med. Educ. Onlin.* **2006**, *11*, 4607. [CrossRef]
32. Masters, K. Preparing Medical Students for the E-Patient. *Med. Teach.* **2017**, *39*, 681–685. [CrossRef]
33. Anthony Berauk, V.L.; Murugiah, M.K.; Soh, Y.C.; Chuan Sheng, Y.; Wong, T.W.; Ming, L.C. Mobile Health Applications for Caring of Older People: Review and Comparison. *Ther. Innov. Regul. Sci.* **2018**, *52*, 374–382. [CrossRef]
34. Masters, K. Artificial Intelligence in Medical Education. *Med. Teach.* **2019**, *41*, 976–980. [CrossRef] [PubMed]
35. Brown Wilson, C.; Slade, C.; Wong, W.Y.A.; Peacock, A. Health Care Students Experience of Using Digital Technology in Patient Care: A Scoping Review of the Literature. *Nurse Educ. Today* **2020**, *95*, 104580. [CrossRef] [PubMed]
36. Hansen, A.; Herrmann, M.; Ehlers, J.P.; Mondritzki, T.; Hensel, K.O.; Truebel, H.; Boehme, P. Perception of the Progressing Digitization and Transformation of the German Health Care System Among Experts and the Public: Mixed Methods Study. *JMIR Public Health Surveill.* **2019**, *5*, e14689. [CrossRef] [PubMed]
37. Mosch, L.; Back, A.; Balzer, F.; Bernd, M.; Brandt, J.; Erkens, S.; Frey, N.; Ghanaat, A.; Glauert, D.L.; Göllner, S.; et al. Lernangebote zu Künstlicher Intelligenz in der Medizin. *Zenodo* **2021**, *1*, 1–86. [CrossRef]
38. Seyhan, A.A.; Carini, C. Are Innovation and New Technologies in Precision Medicine Paving a New Era in Patients Centric Care? *J. Transl. Med.* **2019**, *17*, 114. [CrossRef]
39. Coiera, E. The Price of Artificial Intelligence. *Yearb. Med. Inform.* **2019**, *28*, 14–15. [CrossRef]
40. Bin Dahmash, A.; Alabdulkareem, M.; Alfutais, A.; Kamel, A.M.; Alkholaiwi, F.; Alshehri, S.; Al Zahrani, Y.; Almoaiqel, M. Artificial Intelligence in Radiology: Does It Impact Medical Students Preference for Radiology as Their Future Career? *BJR Open* **2020**, *2*, 20200037. [CrossRef]
41. Reeder, K.; Lee, H. Impact of Artificial Intelligence on US Medical Students' Choice of Radiology. *Clin. Imaging* **2021**, *81*, 67–71. [CrossRef]
42. Webster, C.S. Artificial Intelligence and the Adoption of New Technology in Medical Education. *Med. Educ.* **2021**, *55*, 6–7. [CrossRef]
43. Guadalajara, H.; Palazón, Á.; Lopez-Fernandez, O.; Esteban-Flores, P.; Garcia, J.M.; Gutiérrez-Misis, A.; Baca-García, E.; Garcia-Olmo, D. Towards an Open Medical School without Checkerboards during the COVID-19 Pandemic: How to Flexibly Self-Manage General Surgery Practices in Hospitals? *Healthcare* **2021**, *9*, 743. [CrossRef]

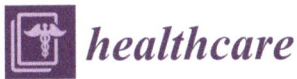

Perspective

Lessons from the COVID-19 Pandemic on the Use of Artificial Intelligence in Digital Radiology: The Submission of a Survey to Investigate the Opinion of Insiders

Daniele Giansanti [1,*], Ivano Rossi [2] and Lisa Monoscalco [3]

1 Centre Tisp, Istituto Superiore di Sanità, 00161 Roma, Italy
2 Faculty of Medicine and Psychology, Sapienza University, Piazzale Aldo Moro, 00185 Roma, Italy; ivano.rossi.univ.sap@gmail.com
3 Faculty of Engineering, Tor Vergata University, Via Cracovia, 00133 Roma, Italy; lisamonoscalco@hotmail.com
* Correspondence: daniele.giansanti@iss.it; Tel.: +39-06-49902701

Citation: Giansanti, D.; Rossi, I.; Monoscalco, L. Lessons from the COVID-19 Pandemic on the Use of Artificial Intelligence in Digital Radiology: The Submission of a Survey to Investigate the Opinion of Insiders. *Healthcare* **2021**, *9*, 331. https://doi.org/10.3390/healthcare9030331

Academic Editor: Tin-Chih Toly Chen

Received: 25 January 2021
Accepted: 10 March 2021
Published: 15 March 2021

Publisher's Note: MDPI stays neutral with regard to jurisdictional claims in published maps and institutional affiliations.

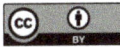

Copyright: © 2021 by the authors. Licensee MDPI, Basel, Switzerland. This article is an open access article distributed under the terms and conditions of the Creative Commons Attribution (CC BY) license (https://creativecommons.org/licenses/by/4.0/).

Abstract: The development of artificial intelligence (AI) during the COVID-19 pandemic is there for all to see, and has undoubtedly mainly concerned the activities of digital radiology. Nevertheless, the strong perception in the research and clinical application environment is that AI in radiology is like a hammer in search of a nail. Notable developments and opportunities do not seem to be combined, now, in the time of the COVID-19 pandemic, with a stable, effective, and concrete use in clinical routine; the use of AI often seems limited to use in research applications. This study considers the future perceived integration of AI with digital radiology after the COVID-19 pandemic and proposes a methodology that, by means of a wide interaction of the involved actors, allows a positioning exercise for acceptance evaluation using a general purpose electronic survey. The methodology was tested on a first category of professionals, the medical radiology technicians (MRT), and allowed to (i) collect their impressions on the issue in a structured way, and (ii) collect their suggestions and their comments in order to create a specific tool for this professional figure to be used in scientific societies. This study is useful for the stakeholders in the field, and yielded several noteworthy observations, among them (iii) the perception of great development in thoracic radiography and CT, but a loss of opportunity in integration with non-radiological technologies; (iv) the belief that it is appropriate to invest in training and infrastructure dedicated to AI; and (v) the widespread idea that AI can become a strong complementary tool to human activity. From a general point of view, the study is a clear invitation to face the last yard of AI in digital radiology, a last yard that depends a lot on the opinion and the ability to accept these technologies by the operators of digital radiology.

Keywords: eHealth; medical devices; mHealth; digital radiology; picture archive and communication system; artificial intelligence; electronic surveys; chest CT; chest radiography

1. Introduction

As for all important diseases, for COVID-19, scholars and scientists have immediately focused on the search for a diagnostic methodology that could give an effective identification response.

Since the first studies related to the appearance of COVID-19, it has been hypothesized that radiography could represent a valid tool [1,2] in the diagnosis of COVID-19 cases. However, it was initially thought that the image alone (therefore, without the application of AI) could not be sufficient due to the possibility of confusion with other pathologies [3]. Scientists and stakeholders moved on to the reverse transcriptase-polymerase chain reaction (abbreviated RT-PCR) [4,5], which was tested and inserted as a gold standard after approval by the CDC and the WHO to identify the virus causing COVID-19. The RT-PCR allows discrimination with other beta-coronaviruses [4,5], and in the context of molecular diagnostics with an appropriate articulated laboratory set-up with certain technical times [6,7], a genomic detection of the virus [8,9].

1.1. Problems with the Use of RT-PCR

This gold standard is not perfect [3], as some studies have reported false negatives [9], and the process is not free from potential errors [10–15].

Furthermore, all health systems are stressed in the use of the gold standard RT-PCR for the following obvious reasons:

1. The big demand is undermining supplies that are very complex due to complex kits and materials to be found during the pandemic.
2. The type of test is particularly expensive due to both the kits and the materials used (the handling difficulties in the COVID-19 era are further increasing in price), both for man time in processing.
3. The reactions involved require important technical times. Time in the pandemic era is showing itself as an important parameter, and is strongly correlated with contact tracing. Longer time implies a higher risk of spreading the SARS-CoV-2 virus.
4. The type of test requires personnel trained in specific degree courses in biomedical laboratory techniques and/or biology.
5. The specific training referred to in the previous point must be done in the presence of others to train the staff in the use of laboratory instruments and kits, and this is very difficult in the pandemic period, since many of the internship activities have been limited and/or replaced with remote activity.
6. Focusing only on a type of test as a gold standard from the point of view of optimization and resource management is required, and an equally effective solution is needed as a backup technique.

We therefore began to seek an answer to the above critical issues by looking with interest towards other solutions. In particular, we began to carefully observe the emerging potential of the world of digital radiology and the world of digital radiology (DR), where the emerging techniques of artificial intelligence, applied to the digital imaging and based on powerful algorithms, seem to have the chance to give important answers point by point to the criticalities reported above.

This is happening in both the X-ray and CT scan sectors.

1.2. Possible at the Moment to Investigate Answers That AI in Digital Radiology Could Give

It is clear that a test system based on AI used in these two sectors shows the following features:

1. It has no supply-critical issues thanks to digital techniques (there are no longer the problems of plate development).
2. It has no material cost problems (for the same reasons as above). In addition, AI can greatly reduce man time with automation.
3. It has a response time that is immediate, which translates into important advantages for contact tracing.
4. It requires trained personnel, but AI automation could make a strong contribution to cost minimization.
5. It needs training, however, the training on diagnostic images can also be practiced through remote techniques thanks to the exchange of images that can also be practiced through telemedicine systems based on eHealth and mHealth.
6. It could represent an alternative and/or backup system.

The development of artificial intelligence (AI) during the COVID-19 pandemic is there for all to see, and has undoubtedly mainly concerned the activities of digital radiology. Since the beginning of the pandemic, the opportunities of AI as a diagnostic tool for COVID-19 through chest CT (CCT) and chest radiography/radiology (CR) have begun to echo.

A simple search on Pubmed with key ((artificial intelligence) AND (chest radiography)) reports 246 studies in 2020 against 131 in 2019, equal to an increase of about 88%. An in-depth analysis with research key ((artificial intelligence) AND (chest radiography) AND (COVID-19) reports that 122 of these articles are focused on or connected to COVID-19.

A search on Pubmed with key ((artificial intelligence) AND (chest CT)) reports 168 studies in 2020 against 59 in 2019, equal to an increase of about 284%. An in-depth analysis with research key ((artificial intelligence) AND (chest CT) AND (COVID-19) reports that 96 of these articles are focused on or connected to COVID-19.

It was also hoped that, through the aforementioned applications, an effective and very fast diagnostic routine and alternative to the gold standard represented by the reverse transcriptase-polymerase chain reaction (abbreviated RT-PCR) technique above reported could be found.

The applications of AI in digital radiology have been remarkable in both sectors of the CCT and CR, as highlighted in wide-ranging reviews by Alsharif et al. [16] and by Ozhain et al. [17]. This was also achieved thanks to the dissemination of large public image databases. Pham in his study reported the usefulness of these databases [18].

In particular, his research is based on three public databases of COVID-19 chest X-rays:

(1) COVID-19 Radiography Database [19],
(2) COVID-19 Chest X-ray Dataset Initiative [20], and
(3) IEEE8023/Covid Chest X-ray Dataset [21].

The first database [18,19] reports both positive and negative images of viral pneumonia. The second database [18–20] reports only full-blown cases of pneumonia due to COVID-19. The third database [18–21] reports positive or suspected cases of viral bacterial pneumonia or COVID-19; besides the radiographic images, it also contains CT images.

As remarked by van Ginneken [22], in this field, numerous specific dedicated architectures have shown exceptional diagnostic performance, such as the DeepCOVID-XR algorithm [23]; CAD4COVID-Xray [?4]; and CV19-Net [25]. The use of three pre-trained convolutional neural networks [18], AlexNet [26], Goog-LeNet [27], and SqueezeNet [28], was shown to be successful by Pham [18]. Many more successful examples of artificial intelligence in this area can be made, although the aim of the work is clearly not to find the best application of AI.

Nevertheless, the strong perception in the research and clinical application environment is that AI in radiology is like a hammer in search of a nail [29]. Notable developments and opportunities do not seem to be combined, now, in the time of the COVID-19 pandemic, with a stable, effective, and concrete use in clinical routine; the use of AI often seems limited to use in research applications. The recurring question is how to raise AI to a more important role in digital radiology, now in a full pandemic, and later at the end of the pandemic.

2. Objective

We have seen that the debate on the use of artificial intelligence during the COVID-19 pandemic is now underway, especially with the focus on the application in digital radiology. We have seen that many recent studies have reported increasing interest on AI in this specific field. Whether and how digital radiology will be affected by the fabulous development achieved by AI during the pandemic is a very important aspect. Surely an important role in this as in many other areas will be played by stakeholders, in our case politicians, territorial governors, and directors of health systems. As mentioned in the editorial [30] dedicated to the special issue entitled The Artificial Intelligence in Digital Pathology and Digital Radiology: Where Are We? opened in the Healthcare (Basel) j, this is one of the classic problems of the last yard of the introduction of AI. Stakeholders have their own sensors on healthcare actors, or at least they should be. The chosen future, the last yard, will depend a lot on the opinion of the actors. An inquiry into their opinion is therefore essential.

It is therefore necessary to focus on AI applied to digital radiology through the two techniques described and to understand the opinion of the users and, in particular, the opinion of the key figures.

In fact, in a top health system, the stakeholders who must direct technological and financial resources must first of all start from the opinion of those who will materially have to work with the renewal of the current process.

In non-pandemic times, a very useful tool was that of meetings with the so-called focus group tool with associations and/or the survey tool.

In a pandemic period, it is almost impossible to develop targeted focus groups, and the survey, perhaps particularly articulated and conducted remotely electronically, can play in addition to the traditional role of collecting opinions (automatically and with the maintenance of social distancing) that of the virtual focus group as well.

The main objective of the study is therefore to:

(a) Develop an electronic survey on this topic suitable for a multitude of healthcare professionals;
(b) Submit it and collect useful suggestions to carry out a specific survey by category useful for subsequent monitoring and interactions with the related scientific companies;
(c) Apply it to a first category of health professionals.

3. Methods

In line with the aim of the study, we decided to develop a survey.
Preliminarily, we have addressed the aspects of privacy and data security.

3.1. Privacy Issues

As the privacy is a very basic issue in submissions of the public surveys we carefully considered this issue.

The questionnaire is anonymous, and the topic did not concern clinical trials on humans, but only opinions and expressions of their thoughts. In consideration of this, it was not considered necessary to proceed with the approval procedures of the EBR.

However, in order to improve the privacy aspects, the workgroup after the suggestion of experts decided not to proceed via e-mail and to avoid requesting the municipality of residence (in small municipalities, this could lead to identification).

We therefore disseminated it capillary through social media, such as Facebook, LinkedIn, Twitter, Instagram, and Whatsapp, association sites, and, in general, using a peer-to-peer dissemination.

3.2. Data Protection Issues

Today, there are several electronic survey applications made available by the great IT giants, such as Microsoft and Google. In this study, Microsoft Forms was chosen, which is available in the Office 365 suite provided to the staff of the Istituto Superiore di Sanità and which for this reason respects the IT security aspects required by current regulations from a systems point of view. Therefore, the tool used for the survey was based solely on resources internal to the system and protected in compliance with the regulations, and has been used in other successful experiences [31–33]. Even if not necessary, since the data in the records are anonymous, the database obtained is managed with care and attention to the data and with the consequent security criteria identified by general rules of best practice in accordance with the legislation.

3.3. Subjects and Perspectives

Regarding the address of the survey, we turned to health personnel.

However, in consideration of the objective of this study and the survey, we also managed the survey as a focus group and developed the following reasoning.

We focused on key figures in interacting with tools and processes and exposure to the Sars-Cov-2 virus. An RT-PCR study would have considered the biomedical lab technician involved in culture preparation and process maintenance as a figure.

Our study has focused more on the figures who legally have to do with radiological processes and have, due to this role, a greater exposure with the virus in the radiology environment.

These figures are those of the medical radiology technicians.

The survey was sent to a large number of subjects, as illustrated in the results, however, the analysis, with the aim of the prospective article, focused on the figure of the medical radiology technician (MRT).

4. Results and Discussion

The first result is represented by the environment with the core element eS.

Figure 1 shows the Quick Response code related to the eS with thefollowing link : https://forms.office.com/Pages/ResponsePage.aspx?id=DQSIkWdsW0yxEjajBLZtrQAAAAAAAAAAAZ_ _gdk7kpUM1JaVENLN01ER0IwWFM0SDdHNjY4TzNKMi4u (accessed on 13 March 2021).

Figure 1. The Quick Response code of the electronic survey.

Figure 2 shows the questions related to the perceived future of AI in DR after the pandemic.

4.1. Numerical Outcome from the Survey

The second result is the outcome from the submission of the eS. At the moment, we have submitted the survey, using the social networks, messaging tools, and other multimedia tools, to a wide sample of 1418 healthcare professionals; among them, 1348 agreed to participate. The submission now is terminated; it lasted from 10 January up to 20 January, and the data analysis will be suitably deepened by means of a specific datamining. Here, with the aim of the perspective overview of the article, we present the outcome from 182 healthcare professionals and medical radiology technicians directly focused in the interaction with the radiology infrastructure. It must also be considered that the survey was designed as a general purpose survey, and with the analysis of the results from the submission on MRTs, as well as validation of the suggestions, was intended to finalize a routine review dedicated to scientific societies.

Figure 3 shows the answers to Likert scale item #16: "Please indicate your opinion on the degree of AI development during the pandemic in the following areas".

Figure 4 shows the answers to the Likert scale item #17: "Indicate in which areas of AI application in radiological diagnostics you would invest after the pandemic".

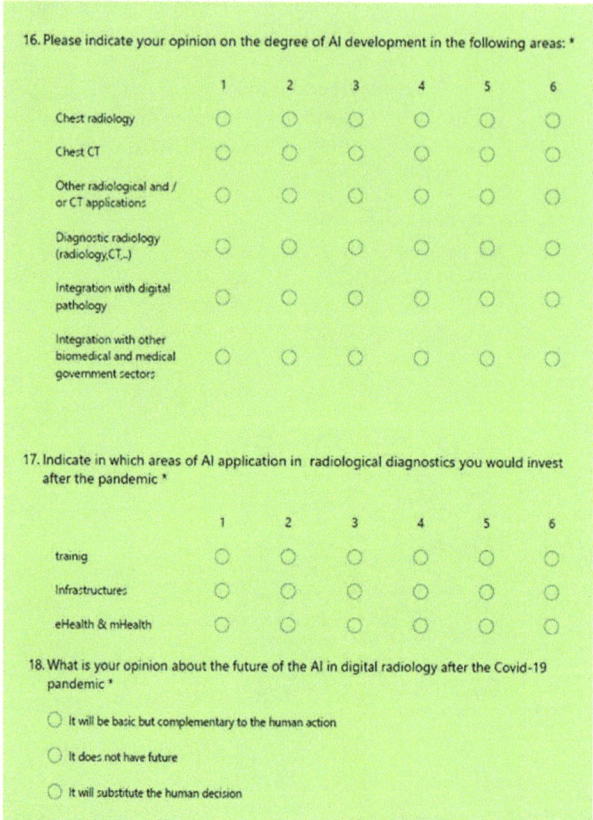

Figure 2. The questions focused on the perceived future of AI after the pandemic N. Q16, Q17, Q18.

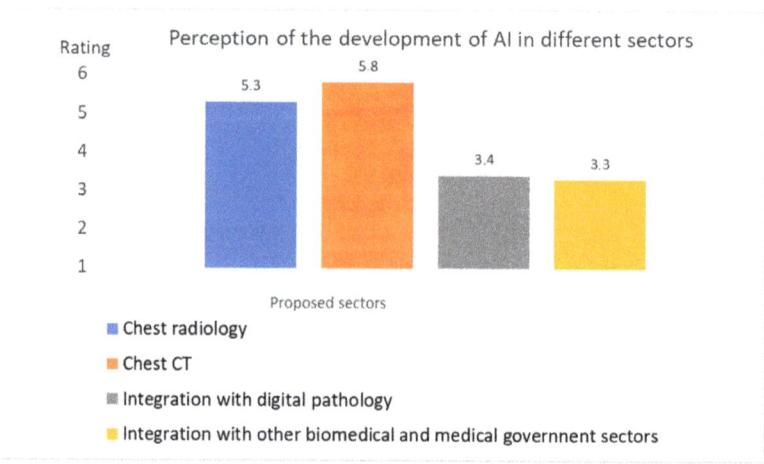

Figure 3. Answers to the Likert scale item #16: "Please indicate your opinion on the degree of AI development during the pandemic in the following areas".

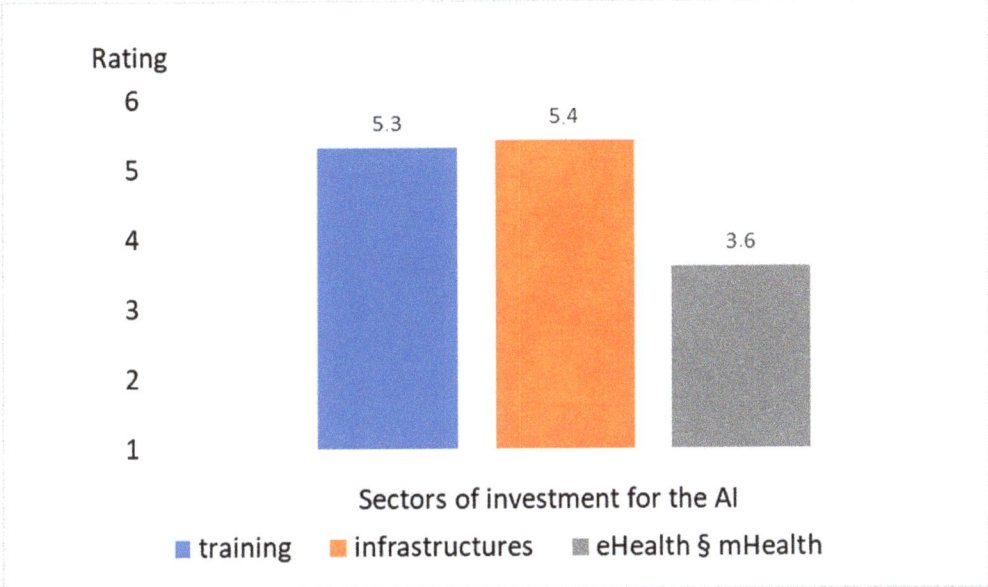

Figure 4. Answers to the Likert scale item #17: "Indicate in which areas of AI application in radiological diagnostics you would invest after the pandemic".

Each question was assigned a score from 1 (min score) to 6 (max score). Therefore, the threshold of agreement (TA) with a proposed aspect was set at 3.5. The outcome from the Likert scale at question #16 (Figure 2) highlighted that:

- Both chest CT and radiography were considered diagnostic areas of great development during the pandemic; both of the average values obtained were higher than TA.
- The other two areas of integration towards other non-radiological technologies were not considered areas of great development, having both obtained a value below the TA threshold.

The results related to the Likert scale at question #17 (Figure 2) highlighted that:

- Both training and infrastructure were considered areas to invest in as far as artificial intelligence is concerned. The values obtained were in fact well above the TA threshold.
- The integration into eHealth and mHealth instead showed a value equal to 3.6, just above the TA threshold.

Figure 5 shows the answers to the multiple choice question #18 (Figure 2): "What is your opinion about the future of AI in digital radiology after the COVID-19 pandemic?" The result showed that, with a very high percentage of 87%, it is believed that AI will make a complementary contribution. Only 10% believed it will replace human decision. Only 3% believed it has no future.

4.2. Validation of the Submission on a Second Sample of MRTs

With the aim of improving and/or proving the validity of the results, we resubmitted the survey to those who did not participate in the first submission in the period from 16 to 21 February 2021 to an independent sample of 98 MRTs. Everyone joined. The repeated analysis in this sample never showed a deviation of more than 1% regarding the values illustrated in the previous analysis. The student *t*-test applied to each pair of mean values of the two submissions never showed significance in the differences between the two mean values.

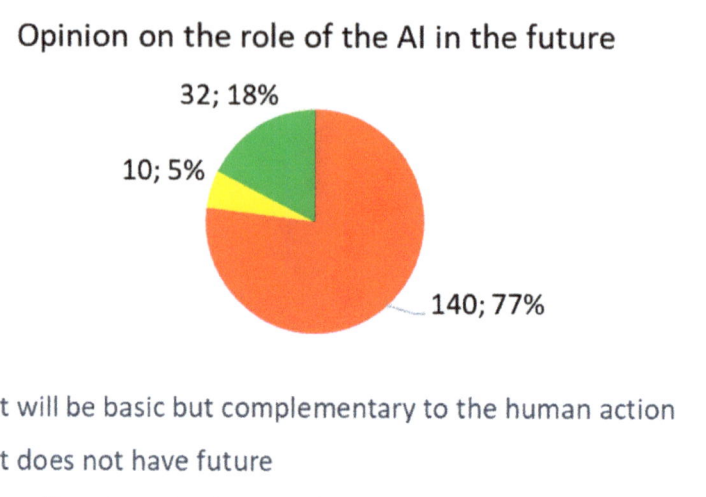

Figure 5. Answers to the multiple choice question #18: "What is your opinion about the future of AI in digital radiology after the COVID-19 pandemic"?

4.3. Comments and Observations from the Survey

As it is visible through the link of the survey, it is possible to insert free comments and observations.

This is importan for collecting through the tool:
(1) Further useful information about the problem.
(2) Observations about the tool itself.

The second point is useful for preparing a further revision of the same survey that will be used several times.

Among the comments (178 in total) that emerged, we found after an interpretative synthesis:

comm-1 Appreciation for the initiative in various forms (150 cases), which then led to the creation of the article. In some cases, the MRT figure was particularly valued.
comm-2 The desire for the survey to be a stable and permanent monitoring tool (11 cases).
comm-3 Concern about the downsizing of one's profession due to possible automatisms (three cases).
comm-4 Lack of confidence in the ability to readjust work processes (four cases) on the basis of AI.
comm-5 The request for further development of the survey on the needs for interaction with AI (in addition to the training one has already foreseen) (four cases).
comm-6 The lack of clarity of the role played in a possible process of interaction with AI (three cases).
comm-7 The clear separation between the world of research and the world of clinical practice in reference to the topic (two cases).
comm-8 The non-usefulness of the questionnaire (one case).

Some of the suggestions and observations collected directly in the survey also emerged in the peer review (see the online reports), and will be used to improve and specialize the tool in the subsequent scheduled submissions specific for the scientific societies of the MRT.

Figure 6 highlights in a logarithmic scale the outcome for each group of comments.

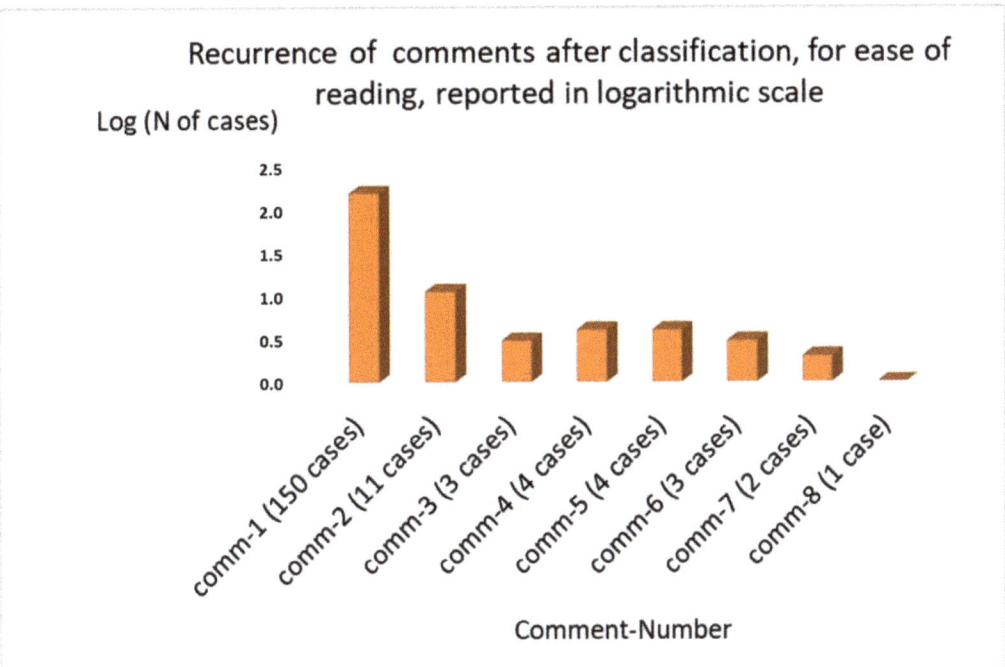

Figure 6. Representation in a logarithmic scale of the comments after the classification.

5. Conclusions and Work in Progress

5.1. Highlights in the Study

Currently, the gold standard in the diagnosis of COVID-19 identified by the CDC and the WHO is RT-PCR [3]. This test in not error free [10–15], and the process is not free from potential errors [18–22]. Furthermore, all health systems are stressed in the use of the gold-standard RT-PCR for the several reasons above described, ranging from the costs to difficulties in supplies. This is pushing scholars and stakeholders to look to other frontiers. The study builds on the frightening developments and the related echo of artificial intelligence in digital radiology [16,17] during the COVID-19 pandemic, and asks questions about the future developments. In particular, it (a) considers the future perceived integration of AI with digital radiology after the COVID-19 pandemic and (b) proposes a solution that, through a mechanism of electronic interaction (protected in the time of COVID-19) with professionals, makes it possible to obtain the opinions and perceptions of a key professional figure in medical radiology processes: the medical radiology technician. This solution, suitably protected regarding the aspects of privacy and data security, made it possible to automatically obtain and process such data for this figure, whose results have been evaluated and discussed, and for other figures whose datamining is continuing. A first added value is the electronic methodology, which has made it possible to prepare a survey in a structured way and in fact also acts as a virtual focus group around the MRT figure. The second added value is represented by the technological solution prepared, which is expandable, even with modifications and specialization (A) both in radiological and other non-radiological realities, such as the world of biomedical laboratory techniques, where AI is also moving, and (B) to other future periods hopefully not marked by the emergency.

The study in general and the data analysis from the survey yielded several noteworthy observations.

From the study clearly emerges the following:

- Digital radiology consists of a management process of radiological techniques and a decision-making process.
- The heart of the management process is the MRT, who interacts with the patient in the radiology laboratory and who is also the figure most exposed to COVID-19.
- Certainly, artificial intelligence could simplify processes with automation, reducing processing times (including exposure), decision times, and costs.
- Training in packages dedicated to AI applied to radiology could also be done with tutorials and remote training and exercises carried out on large public databases available, such as those shown in the study.
- The massive use of eHealth and/or mHealth solutions could make it easier to interact and finalize the further decision-making and/or administrative processes of RIS and HIS.

From the survey clearly emerges from the closed questions:

- The perception of a great development in thoracic radiography and CT, but a loss of opportunity in integration with non-radiological technologies.
- The belief that it is appropriate to invest in training and infrastructure dedicated to AI.
- The widespread idea that AI can become a strong complementary tool to human activity.

We also deepened the open questions in a dedicated final space of the survey, from which the appreciation for the initiative in various forms (which then led to the creation of the article) for the highlighting the role of the MRT figure and the desire that the tool become stable for future initiatives were most evident. In a few cases, this outcome highlights (i) the concern about the downsizing of one's profession due to possible automatisms, and (ii) the lack of confidence in the ability to readjust work processes on the basis of AI. From this analysis (iii) some useful suggestions were also highlighted (starting from the general purpose survey) from a specialist survey focused on MRT to be used by scientific societies.

From a general point of view, the study is a clear invitation to face the last yard of AI in digital radiology, an important issue that depends a lot on the opinion and the ability to accept these technologies by the operators of digital radiology.

5.2. Work in Progress

From a general point of view, the questionnaire was a general purpose tool intended for a wide category of professionals. In this study, the outcome of a category of strategic professionals in digital radiology, that of MRTs, was evaluated. From this outcome and the review process, important considerations and suggestions emerged for the finalization of a specific tool for this figure to be used in scientific societies. The link below allows you to access and see some specializations prepared, and see the survey currently: https://forms.office.com/Pages/ResponsePage.aspx?id=DQSIkWdsW0yxEjajBLZtrQAAAAAAAAAAAZ__gdk7kpUQ001Nk5ORDVPMjk0M0g4RkdPQkdOOUwwSi4u (accessed on 13 March 2021).

Figure 7 shows a print screen of some changes made that allow, through two sets of multiple choice questions and two open questions, to investigate aspects of this figure's wishes and expectations towards AI.

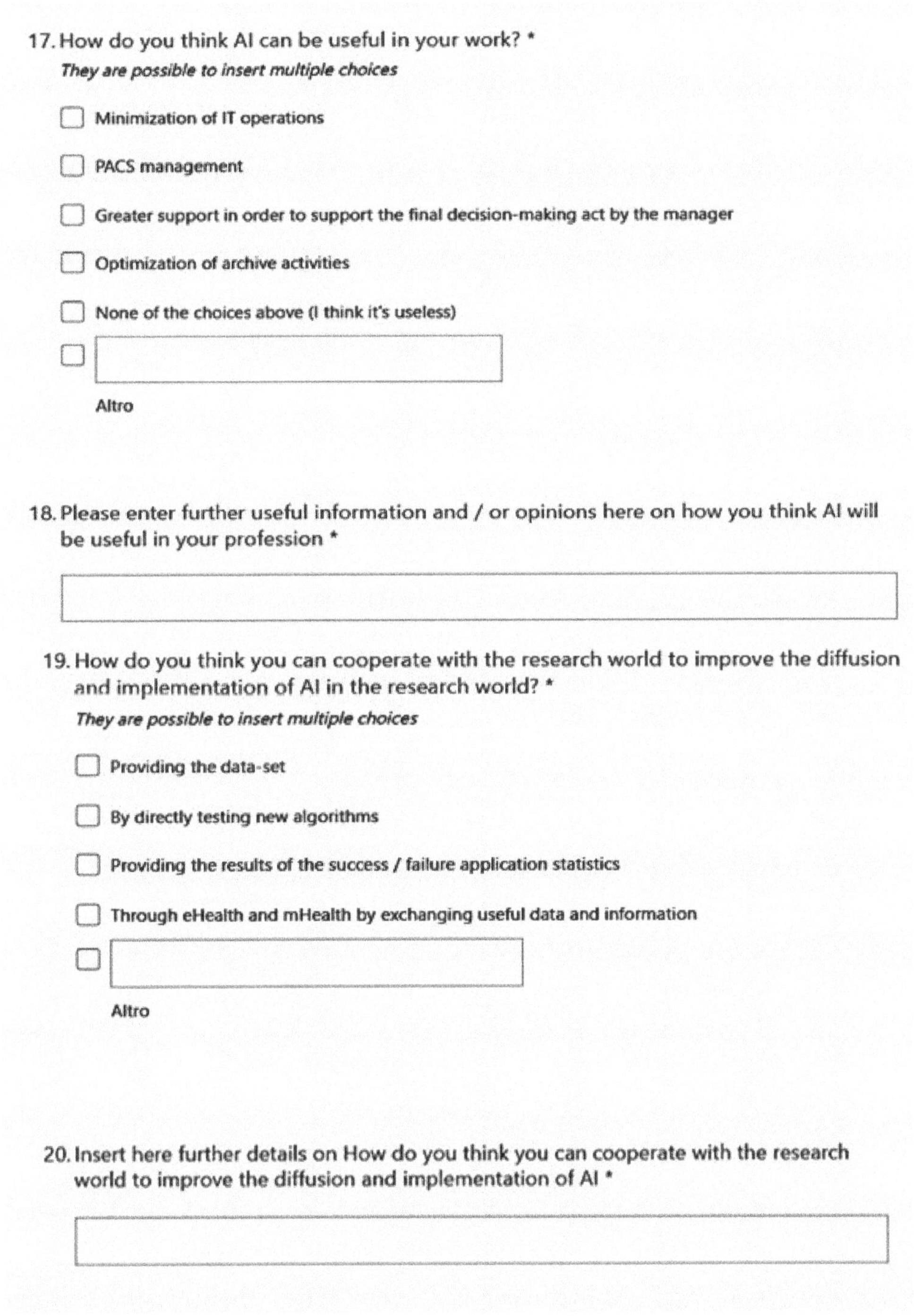

17. How do you think AI can be useful in your work? *
    They are possible to insert multiple choices

    ☐ Minimization of IT operations

    ☐ PACS management

    ☐ Greater support in order to support the final decision-making act by the manager

    ☐ Optimization of archive activities

    ☐ None of the choices above (I think it's useless)

    ☐ [_____]
    Altro

18. Please enter further useful information and / or opinions here on how you think AI will be useful in your profession *

    [_____]

19. How do you think you can cooperate with the research world to improve the diffusion and implementation of AI in the research world? *
    They are possible to insert multiple choices

    ☐ Providing the data-set

    ☐ By directly testing new algorithms

    ☐ Providing the results of the success / failure application statistics

    ☐ Through eHealth and mHealth by exchanging useful data and information

    ☐ [_____]
    Altro

20. Insert here further details on How do you think you can cooperate with the research world to improve the diffusion and implementation of AI *

    [_____]

Figure 7. Some sections inserted in the specialized tool for the MRTs focused on the usefulness of AI in the MRT profession and the idea of cooperation of MRTs with the world of research in the field of AI.

Author Contributions: Conceptualization, D.G.; methodology, D.G.; software, all; validation, all; formal analysis, all; investigation, all; resources, D.G.; data curation, D.G.; writing—original draft preparation, D.G.; writing—review and editing, all; supervision, D.G.; project administration, D.G. All authors have read and agreed to the published version of the manuscript.

Funding: This research received no external funding.

Institutional Review Board Statement: Not applicable.

Informed Consent Statement: Not applicable.

Data Availability Statement: Data sharing not applicable.

Conflicts of Interest: The authors declare no conflict of interest.

References

1. Fu, L.; Wang, B.; Yuan, T.; Chen, X.; Ao, Y.; Fitzpatrick, T.; Li, P.; Zhou, Y.; Lin, Y.F.; Duan, Q.; et al. Clinical characteristics of coronavirus disease 2019 (COVID-19) in China: A systematic review and meta-analysis. *J. Infect.* **2020**, *80*, 656–665. [CrossRef] [PubMed]
2. Huang, C.; Wang, Y.; Li, X.; Ren, L.; Zhao, J.; Hu, Y.; Zhang, L.; Fan, G.; Xu, J.; Gu, X.; et al. Clinical features of patients infected with 2019 novel coronavirus in Wuhan, China. *Lancet* **2020**, *395*, 497–506. [CrossRef]
3. Rahbari, R.; Moradi, N.; Abdi, M. rRT-PCR for SARS-CoV-2: Analytical considerations. *Clin. Chim. Acta* **2021**, *516*, 1–7. [CrossRef] [PubMed]
4. Corman, V.M.; Landt, O.; Kaiser, M.; Molenkamp, R.; Meijer, A.; Chu, D.K.; Bleicker, T.; Brunink, S.; Schneider, J.; Schmidt, M.L.; et al. Detection of 2019 novel coronavirus (2019-nCoV) by real-time RT-PCR. *Eurosurveillance* **2020**, *25*, 2000045. [CrossRef] [PubMed]
5. Pang, J.; Wang, M.X.; Ang, I.Y.H.; Tan, S.H.X.; Lewis, R.F.; Chen, J.I.; Gutierrez, R.A.; Gwee, S.X.W.; Chua, P.E.Y.; Yang, Q.; et al. Potential Rapid Diagnostics, Vaccine and Therapeutics for 2019 Novel Coronavirus (2019-nCoV): A Systematic Review. *J. Clin. Med.* **2020**, *9*, 623. [CrossRef] [PubMed]
6. Kaltenboeck, B.; Wang, C. Advances in real-time PCR: Application to clinical laboratory diagnostics. *Adv. Clin. Chem.* **2005**, *40*, 219–259. [PubMed]
7. Mayer, G.; Muller, J.; Lunse, C.E. RNA diagnostics: Real-time RT-PCR strategies and promising novel target RNAs. *Wiley Interdiscip. Rev. RNA* **2011**, *2*, 32–41. [CrossRef] [PubMed]
8. Jin, Y.H.; Cai, L.; Cheng, Z.S.; Cheng, H.; Deng, T.; Fan, Y.P.; Fang, C.; Huang, D.; Huang, L.Q.; Huang, Q.; et al. A rapid advice guideline for the diagnosis and treatment of 2019 novel coronavirus (2019-nCoV) infected pneumonia (standard version). *Mil. Med. Res.* **2020**, *7*, 4. [CrossRef]
9. Lippi, G.; Plebani, M. Laboratory abnormalities in patients with COVID-2019 infection. *Clin. Chem. Lab. Med.* **2020**, *58*, 1131–1134. [CrossRef] [PubMed]
10. Lippi, G.; Simundic, A.M.; Plebani, M. Potential preanalytical and analytical vulnerabilities in the laboratory diagnosis of coronavirus disease 2019 (COVID-19). *Clin. Chem. Lab. Med.* **2020**, *58*, 1070–1076. [CrossRef]
11. Espy, M.J.; Uhl, J.R.; Sloan, L.M.; Buckwalter, S.P.; Jones, M.F.; Vetter, E.A.; Yao, J.D.; Wengenack, N.L.; Rosenblatt, J.E.; Smith, F.; et al. Real-time PCR in clinical microbiology: Applications for routine laboratory testing. *Clin. Microbiol. Rev.* **2006**, *19*, 165–256. [CrossRef] [PubMed]
12. Lippi, G.; Lima-Oliveira, G.; Brocco, G.; Bassi, A.; Salvagno, G.L. Estimating the intra- and inter-individual imprecision of manual pipetting. *Clin. Chem. Lab. Med.* **2017**, *55*, 962–966. [CrossRef] [PubMed]
13. Lippi, G.; von Meyer, A.; Cadamuro, J.; Simundic, A.M.C. European Federation of Clinical, P. Laboratory Medicine Working Group for Preanalytical, PREDICT: A checklist for preventing preanalytical diagnostic errors in clinical trials. *Clin. Chem. Lab. Med.* **2020**, *58*, 518–526. [CrossRef]
14. van Zyl, G.; Maritz, J.; Newman, H.; Preiser, W. Lessons in diagnostic virology: Expected and unexpected sources of error. *Rev. Med. Virol.* **2019**, *29*, e2052. [PubMed]
15. Tang, Y.W.; Schmitz, J.E.; Persing, D.H.; Stratton, C.W. Laboratory Diagnosis of COVID-19: Current Issues and Challenges. *J. Clin. Microbiol.* **2020**, *58*, 108. [CrossRef]
16. Alsharif, M.H.; Alsharif, Y.H.; Yahya, K.; Alomari, O.A.; Albreem, M.A.; Jahid, A. Deep learning applications to combat the dissemination of COVID-19 disease: A review. *Eur. Rev. Med. Pharmacol. Sci.* **2020**, *24*, 11455–11460. [CrossRef]
17. Ozsahin, I.; Sekeroglu, B.; Musa, M.S.; Mustapha, M.T.; Uzun Ozsahin, D. Review on Diagnosis of COVID-19 from Chest CT Images Using Artificial Intelligence. *Comput. Math. Methods Med.* **2020**, *2020*, 9756518. [CrossRef]
18. Pham, T.D. Classification of COVID-19 chest X-rays with deep learning: New models or fine tuning? *Health Inf. Sci. Syst.* **2020**, *9*, 2. [CrossRef]
19. COVID-19 Radiography Database. Available online: https://www.kaggle.com/tawsifurrahman/covid19-radiography-database (accessed on 2 July 2020).

20. COVID-19 Chest X-ray Dataset Initiative. Available online: https://github.com/agchung/Figure1-COVID-chestxray-dataset (accessed on 2 July 2020).
21. IEEE8023/Covid Chest X-ray Dataset. Available online: https://github.com/ieee8023/covid-chestxray-dataset (accessed on 2 July 2020).
22. van Ginneken, B. The Potential of Artificial Intelligence to Analyze Chest Radiographs for Signs of COVID-19 Pneumonia. *Radiology* **2020**, 204238. [CrossRef]
23. Wehbe, R.M.; Sheng, J.; Dutta, S.; Chai, S.; Dravid, A.; Barutcu, S.; Wu, Y.; Cantrell, D.R.; Xiao, N.; Allen, B.D.; et al. DeepCOVID-XR: An Artificial Intelligence Algorithm to Detect COVID-19 on Chest Radiographs Trained and Tested on a Large US Clinical Dataset. *Radiology* **2020**, 203511. [CrossRef]
24. Murphy, K.; Smits, H.; Knoops, A.J.G.; Korst, M.B.J.M.; Samson, T.; Scholten, E.T.; Schalekamp, S.; Schaefer-Prokop, C.M.; Philipsen, R.H.H.M.; Meijers, A.; et al. COVID-19 on the Chest Radiograph: A Multi-Reader Evaluation of an AI System. *Radiology* **2020**, *296*, E166–E172. [CrossRef]
25. Zhang, R.; Xin Tie, X.; Qi, Z.; Bevins, N.B.; Zhang, C.; Griner, D.; Song, T.K.; Nadig, J.D.; Schiebler, M.L.; Garrett, J.W.; et al. Diagnosis of COVID-19 Pneumonia Using Chest Radiography: Value of Artificial Intelligence. *Radiology* **2020**. [CrossRef]
26. Krizhevsky, A.; Sutskever, I.; Hinton, G.E. ImageNet classification with deep convolutional neural networks. *Commun. ACM* **2017**, *60*, 84–90. [CrossRef]
27. Szegedy, C.; Liu, W.; Jia, Y.; Sermanet, P.; Reed, S.; Anguelov, D.; Erhan, D.; Vanhoucke, V.; Rabinovich, A. Going deeper with convolutions. In Proceedings of the IEEE Conference on Computer Vision and Pattern Recognition, Columbus, OH, USA, 23–28 June 2015; pp. 1–9.
28. Iandola, F.N.; Han, S.; Moskewicz, M.W.; Ashraf, K.; Dally, W.J.; Keutzer, K. SqueezeNet: AlexNet-level accuracy with 50x fewer parameters and <0.5 MB model size. *arXiv* **2016**, arXiv:1602.07360.
29. Summers, R.M. Artificial Intelligence of COVID-19 Imaging: A Hammer in Search of a Nail. *Radiology* **2020**, 204226. [CrossRef]
30. Giansanti, D. The artificial intelligence in digital pathology and digital radiology: Where are we? *Healthcare* **2021**, *9*, 30. [CrossRef]
31. Giansanti, D. Towards the evolution of the mHealth in mental health with youth: The cyber-space used in psychological rehabilitation is becoming wearable into a pocket. *mHealth* **2020**, *6*, 18. [CrossRef] [PubMed]
32. Giansanti, D.; Monoscalco, L. The Cyber-Risk in Cardiology: Towards an Investigation on the Self Perception among the Cardiologists. *mHealth* **2020**. Available online: https://mhealth.amegroups.com/article/view/37310/28600 (accessed on 13 March 2021).
33. Giansanti, D.; Monoscalco, L. A smartphone-based survey in mHealth to investigate the introduction of the artificial intelligence into cardiology. *mHealth* **2021**. [CrossRef] [PubMed]

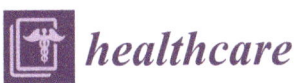 healthcare

Review

The Artificial Intelligence in Digital Radiology: Part 1: The Challenges, Acceptance and Consensus

Daniele Giansanti [1,*] and Francesco Di Basilio [2]

1. Centro Tisp, Istituto Superiore di Sanità, 00161 Roma, Italy
2. Facoltà di Medicina e Psicologia, Università Sapienza, 00185 Roma, Italy; fdibasilio@hotmail.com
* Correspondence: daniele.giansanti@iss.it; Tel.: +39-06-49902701

Abstract: Artificial intelligence is having important developments in the world of digital radiology also thanks to the boost given to the research sector by the COVID-19 pandemic. In the last two years, there was an important development of studies focused on both challenges and acceptance and consensus in the field of Artificial Intelligence. The challenges and acceptance and consensus are two strategic aspects in the development and integration of technologies in the health domain. The study conducted two narrative reviews by means of two parallel points of view to take stock both on the ongoing challenges and on initiatives conducted to face the acceptance and consensus in this area. The methodology of the review was based on: (I) search of PubMed and Scopus and (II) an eligibility assessment, using parameters with 5 levels of score. The results have: (a) highlighted and categorized the important challenges in place. (b) Illustrated the different types of studies conducted through original questionnaires. The study suggests for future research based on questionnaires a better calibration and inclusion of the challenges in place together with validation and administration paths at an international level.

Keywords: digital radiology; radiology; picture archive and communication system; artificial intelligence

1. Introduction

We are witnessing the introduction of Artificial Intelligence in many areas of medicine. Among these sectors, we find the sector of digital radiology and digital pathology. The potential is very large. Although with different speeds and degrees of use, Artificial Intelligence is proving useful in both sectors in many activities. The radiology and pathology *workflow* can certainly benefit from a routine use of Artificial Intelligence. The advantages that could derive from this seem important [1]. They range from lightening the workload to quality control of the instrumentation. The hospital routine, however, has some mandatory steps before the implementation. Among these passages, we certainly find those relating to *acceptance* and *consensus*. The *acceptance* and *consensus*, with regards to the Artificial Intelligence, are playing an increasing interest both in Digital Radiology and Digital Pathology and are among the topics of strong attention of the Special Issue "The Artificial Intelligence in Digital Pathology and Digital Radiology: Where Are We?" [2].

The recent experience of Artificial Intelligence in Digital Radiology, during the still active pandemic, seems promising. The successful applications of Artificial Intelligence in Chest Computerized Tomography/Radiography seem to bring the moment of the introduction in the clinical routine ever closer [3,4].

This will certainly happen through an adequate transfer of Evidence-Based Medicine to clinical practice and the *health domain, by means of agreement tools*. The Technology Assessment tools, such as the Health Technology Assessment and the comparative effectiveness research [5], will certainly be useful. Other methodologies, such as the Consensus Conference methodologies [6], will be able to be implemented. Consensus Conferences are currently used successfully in other emerging sectors using also Artificial Intelligence such as Robotics [7,8]. From future studies, useful guidelines for clinical dissemination will presumably emerge [9].

Artificial Intelligence is subject to continuous challenges in the integration process within the *health domain* [10]. To face a good process of integrating Artificial Intelligence with Digital Radiology, it is necessary first: (a) to always creating new challenges "separating Hope from Hype" and avoiding pitfalls [10]; (b) to ensure that processes of acceptance and consensus of the insiders accompany these challenges, who will have to do with these technologies in their *workflow*. Therefore, the challenges will have to be followed by integration processes in the *health domain*, by means of agreement tools based also on studies of *acceptance and consensus*.

2. Purpose

The purpose of the study was to focus on the Artificial Intelligence integration and:

(a) To examine the main challenges in the field in relation to integration in the health domain. This point is addressed to answer the key question *"What are the current challenges to be faced in integrating these technologies into the health domain?"*
(b) To deal with the topic of acceptance in the health domain and to address the relevant state of implementation of the used tools to assess this on the insiders. This point is addressed to answer the key question *"What tools are currently used to evaluate the acceptance of these technologies among insiders?"*
(c) As a side objective, to analyse how the challenges and acceptance are connected to each other and what are the possible ways to proceed to improve the integration of consensus among insiders. This point is addressed to answer the key question *"What suggestions emerge from the study to improve the tools used to assess acceptance among insiders, in light of what emerges in the previous points?"*

3. Methods

According to the purpose, the study faced the three points of view.

Regarding the search of the studies, we considered that all points address the integration in the health domain. Therefore, we decided to orient ourselves first of all towards a database that contains international peer-reviewed studies in this area.

We also considered the interdisciplinary aspects of the topic and we thought that the search had to be deepened also using a multidisciplinary database, always considering that the selection of the articles (see below) had to strongly consider the integration in the health domain. We have chosen PubMed (an archive focusing primarily on the life sciences and biomedical disciplines that contains Medline) as our main database. We have also expanded our search to include Scopus, a multidisciplinary database; however, strictly considering that we dealt with aspects of the health domain.

The first two points faced literature searches, with targeted keys and through an eligibility process. The eligibility process was based on a scoring system (with different parameters and a score with 5 levels) applied by the two experts (plus one adjudicator in case of discordance), to include each reference. It is possible to assign a score to these parameters ranging from a minimum score of one (minimum) up to a maximum of five (maximun). Table 1 shows the scoring system.

The study was excluded, regardless of the score, if there were critical issues of conflict of interest (for example, it was conducted without guarantees of objectivity by the system manufacturer).

The study was included in the review if all parameters were scored ≥ 3.0.

The third point is a point of reflection, based on what emerges in the previous points, and therefore faced in the discussion.

The specific searches for the first two points are:

(First point of view) Search has been carried out in this area considering the key in Table 2.

Table 1. Parameters used for the qualification.

Parameter	Description	Score (1 = min; 5 = max)
1	Is the research design appropriate?	
2	Are the methods adequately described?	
3	Are the results clearly presented?	
4	Are the conclusions supported by results	
5	Added contribute to the field	
6	Topicality level of the study	
7	Focus on the health domain	

Table 2. Keys used in the search (also with plurals).

Key
"artificial intelligence"[Title/Abstract] AND "radiology"[Title/Abstract] AND ("challenges"[Title/Abstract] OR "future research"[Title/Abstract] OR "integration"[Title/Abstract] OR "opportunity"[Title/Abstract] OR "future direction"[Title/Abstract])

(Second point of view) Search has been carried out in this area considering the keys in Table 3.

Table 3. Keys used in the search related to the second point of view (also with plurals).

Key
"artificial intelligence"[Title/Abstract] AND ("radiology"[MeSH Terms] OR "radiology"[All Fields] OR "radiography"[MeSH Terms] OR "radiography"[All Fields] OR "radiology s"[All Fields]) AND ("accept"[All Fields] OR "acceptabilities"[All Fields] OR "acceptability"[All Fields] OR "acceptable"[All Fields] OR "acceptably"[All Fields] OR "acceptance"[All Fields] OR "acceptances"[All Fields] OR "acceptation"[All Fields] OR "accepted"[All Fields] OR "accepter"[All Fields] OR "accepters"[All Fields] OR "accepting"[All Fields] OR "accepts"[All Fields])
("consensual"[All Fields] OR "consensually"[All Fields] OR "consensus"[MeSH Terms] OR "consensus"[All Fields]) AND "artificial intelligence"[Title/Abstract] AND "radiology"[Title/Abstract]

4. Results

4.1. The Challenges

In line with the first objective of the study, we analysed the main challenges in the design and integration of Artificial Intelligence in digital radiology. The eligibility process led to the choice of 20 papers [11–30], among which there are mainly reviews (15 in number) (as it could be expected considering the broad topics covered) but also 5 recent scientific articles/focus articles on very specific aspects [15,26,27,29,30].

The search highlighted how:

- The picture that emerged was that of a scientific production touching all aspects relating to the challenges, from the challenges on algorithms [13] up to challenges on the ethical and legal issues [14].
- These challenges according to the following thematic analysis are arranged into six paragraphs with the synopsis of each paper.

4.1.1. Challenges on Algorithms

A first study by Fazal et al. [11], on this topic, was relating to the evolution and perspectives of use of algorithms. The study showed that, after an initial difficulty, due to the limitation of the technology in 1960, the introduction of Artificial Intelligence-based computer-aided detection software in the 1980s marked the advent of widespread integration of Artificial Intelligence within radiology reporting. The authors pointed out among the macro areas of challenges in the algorithms: (a) to decrease the false-positive rates causing a limitation for computer-aided detection, although this has strongly improved.

(b) The better understanding of the Artificial Intelligence reasoning: (c) The well definition of responsibility in case of the error caused by the algorithms.

Another study by Maowad et al. [12] specifically focused on the challenges of machine learning and deep learning, subclasses of Artificial Intelligence that showed breakthrough performance in image analysis. The authors discussed the current applications of machine learning and deep learning in the field of diagnostic radiology. They highlighted that deep learning applications could be divided into medical imaging analysis and applications beyond analysis. The authors also highlighted how beyond image analysis, deep learning could be used for quality control, workflow organization, and reporting revolutionizing the activity of the insiders.

The study by Barragan-Montero et al. [27] faced the challenges for a safe and efficient use of clinical Artificial Intelligence applications. They reported that this depended, in part, on informed practitioners and reviewed the pillars of Artificial Intelligence, together with state-of-the-art machine learning methods and their application to medical imaging.

They metaphorically depicted that artificial intelligence, machine learning, and deep learning could be seen as *matryoshkas* nested in each other. Artificial intelligence gathered both symbolic (top–down) and connectionist (bottom–up) approaches. Machine learning was the dominant branch of connectionism, combining biological (neural networks) and statistical (data-driven learning theory) influences. Deep learning focused mainly on large-size neural networks, with functional specificities to process images. According to this, they reported a very fine mapping between different learning frameworks and strategies (together with some of the most popular algorithms or techniques used for each of them) and specific medical applications, tabling in details. This mapping was divided into three parts in the tabling: the basic learning frameworks (supervised, unsupervised and reinforcement learning); the hybrid learning frameworks blending supervised and unsupervised; and finally, common learning strategies solving consecutive learning problems or combining several models together.

4.1.2. Challenges Focused on the Professionalism of the Radiologist

These innovations of Artificial Intelligence in Digital Radiology mainly revolve around the professional aspects of the radiologist.

The study by Gampala el al. [16] highlighted the challenges around this professional at the end of the medical decision chain. Artificial Intelligence could simplify every activity, like ordering and scheduling, protocoling and acquisition, image interpretation, reporting, communication, and billing. Therefore, Artificial Intelligence could be useful both in the diagnosis (supporting the categorization activities with the image enhancement, feature assessment and recognition) and in the patient management and workflow. Therefore, the same way physicians were familiar with planning protocols or delineation guidelines, the clinical teams should start being familiar with guiding principles for data management and curation in the era of Artificial Intelligence.

In line with this study, the study by Barragan-Montero et al. [27] highlighted how the Findability, Accessibility, Interoperability, and Reusability Data Principles [27] used in digital radiology must be rethought through challenges around the radiologist, including Artificial Intelligence.

The readjustment of these principles, according to the study by Banja et al. [26], encounters major challenges [26] regarding ethical and regulatory implications in the development and use of algorithms. All three studies [16,26,27] showed in a complementary way how, to support the radiologist, data science specialists should work on the development of increasingly performing and targeted algorithms, calibrated considering the specificity of the application, the decision-making protocols, and the physical process, which is different from time to time in the formation of images. For this reason, it is important that the radiologist talks with these scientific professionals, also involved in basic research, both to give new stimuli and to give feedback on use.

4.1.3. Challenges on the Tools, Datasets, and the Workflow

The challenges in Digital Radiology were also mentioned in the study by Ahmad [17], in the study by Hamed et al. [18], and in the study by Kottler [19]. Particular emphasis was dedicated to the challenges in the engineering and in the machine in terms of hardware, software, and impact on the workflow. These studies [17–19] also reported important new activities such as selecting Artificial Intelligence products and vendors; piloting vendors' Artificial Intelligence algorithms; creating our own Artificial Intelligence algorithms; implementing, optimizing, and maintaining these algorithms.

The study by Martin-Noguerol et al. [20] specifically focused on the challenges on the tools development. It reported the importance of the tools for the *use cases* and described them, including clinical registries, tools validation, and assistance for radiology reporting. In details, they reported a review of the tools required for successful implementation of the use cases.

The study by Cushnan et al. [28] emphasized the importance of the *use cases* and the experience of the National COVID-19 Chest Imaging Database, led by the British Society of Thoracic Imaging, Royal Surrey National Health Service Foundation Trust and Faculty in the collection of datasets on a national scale. This was a challenging experience to execute for several reasons, including issues with data privacy, the lack of data reporting standards, interoperable technologies, and distribution methods. The authors reported that this is a key issue to advance the safe adoption of artificial intelligence in the health domain.

4.1.4. Challenges on the Teamwork

A wide-range teamwork should work on the Artificial Intelligence development in digital radiology. The study by Martin-Noguerol et al. [20] reported the challenges in teamwork around these tools and, in particular, in the collaboration between engineers, systems developers and radiologists. The communication between radiologists and data scientists was considered crucial for successful collaborative work. There were emphasized the specific skills that are inherent to radiological and medical training, critical for identifying anatomical or clinical targets as well as for segmenting or labelling lesions. According to the authors, these skills would then have to be transferred, explained, and taught to the data science experts to facilitate their comprehension and integration algorithms. The study by Pesapane et al. [21] reported how the role of the stakeholders was also considered strategic in this team game. The authors reported that the stakeholders had the opinion that Artificial Intelligence could improve the practice of radiology and that they considered the replacement of radiologists unlikely. Furthermore, the study reported that stakeholders identified the need for education and training on Artificial Intelligence, as well as collaborative efforts to improve Artificial Intelligence implementation.

4.1.5. Challenges on the Education

The education and training were considered key factors for the integration of Artificial Intelligence in the health domain in different studies [15,22,23,29,30].

The study by Pesapane et al. [22] highlighted that the training needed to be continuous, specialized and based on a strong mobility on the territory, because it had to consider the continuous evolution of Artificial Intelligence.

The study by Pianiykh et al. [23] stressed the importance of continuous training, taking into account that network-based algorithms follow continuous learning processes [23]. The study by Fischetti et al. [30] showed how, with the integration of artificial intelligence within medicine, it was likely that the current medical trainee curricula could experience the impact it had to offer both for education and for medical practice. The study deepened the landscape of radiologic education within the current medical trainee curricula, and faced how artificial intelligence could potentially influence the current and future radiologic education model. From a specular point of view, the study by Reeder et al. [15] highlighted how Artificial Intelligence could also have a negative impact on the university choice of students. It underlined that Artificial Intelligence had a significantly negative impact on American medical students' choice of radiology as a career, a phenomenon influenced by both individual concerns and exposure to Artificial Intelligence from the medical community. According to these authors, the challenge was also to avoid the impact of misinformation on Artificial Intelligence. In line with this, the study by Morrison et al. [29] reported the importance of education together with greater clarity of language. They concluded this by means of a thematic analysis that considered both the education and the clarity of language as favourable factors for eliminating the barriers to the adoption of Artificial Intelligence in the National Health Service.

4.1.6. Challenges on the Ethical and Regulatory Issues

Among the challenges, there were also those of the impact of ethical aspects [14,24,25] and of legal regulation [14,25]. In fact, with the growth in the use of Artificial Intelligence as a medical device, alone or interconnected with the network, the adaptation and compliance with the legislation was considered a fundamental challenge in terms of all aspects of use in the free market.

The study by Pesapane et al. [14] analysed the regulation in the context of medical device development, and the challenges to make Artificial Intelligence applications safe and useful in the future. The authors analysed the legal framework regulating medical devices and data protection in Europe and in the United States. The European Union was reforming these fields with new legislation (General Data Protection Regulation, Cybersecurity Directive, Medical Devices Regulation, In Vitro Diagnostic Medical Device Regulation). As regards the United States, the Food and Drug Administration predominantly controlled the regulatory scene. The study highlighted these fundamental aspects: -Artificial Intelligence applications were medical devices supporting detection/diagnosis, workflow, cost-effectiveness. -Regulations for safety, privacy protection, and ethical use of sensitive information were needed. -Europe and the United States had different approaches for approving and regulating new medical devices. -European laws considered cyberattacks, incidents (notification and minimisation), and service continuity. -Laws in the United Sates asked for opt-in data processing and use as well as for clear consumer consent. The study by Jaremko et al. [25] provided a framework for study of the legal and ethical issues on Artificial Intelligence in medical imaging, related to patient data (privacy, confidentiality, ownership, and sharing); algorithms (levels of autonomy, liability, and jurisprudence); practice (best practices and current legal framework); and finally, opportunities in Artificial Intelligence from the perspective of a universal healthcare system. The study by Akinci et al. [24] was entirely devoted to ethical aspects in radiology applications. The ethical issues were discussed under the light of core biomedical ethics principles and principles for Artificial Intelligence specific ethical challenges, while giving an overview of the statements that were proposed for the ethics of Artificial Intelligence applications in radiology.

4.2. The Tools Used to Assess the Acceptance

In line with the second objective of the study, we analysed the acceptance in the integration into the health domain. Many studies were excluded after a first rapid screening since the specific keys of research (e.g., acceptance) were not associated with content developed on this topic, and/or were associated with other contexts and/or cited in a single occurrence in a sentence.

After this quick first screening, the eligibility process led to the choice of 15 papers [31–44].

The analysis was arranged into two paragraphs. The first one reports the general considerations that emerge in these studies. The second one reports a detailed analysis with the synopsis of each paper.

4.2.1. General Considerations on the Tools for the Acceptance

The search highlighted:
(a) that the selected papers showed that the tools were essentially based on questionnaires [31–44];
(b) that the interest into this theme is recent, since publications of studies have started very recently, as the first ones are from 2019, and this reinforces the need for this study.

The selected papers [31–44] showed that the studies focused on some of the actors in this area: radiologists, radiographers, primary care providers, developers, students, and patients, that is, on both service providers and users, and on the subjects in training.

In some cases, comparative studies were carried out on the different actors.

Surveys were used to collect both interviews and structured data. In all identified cases, questionnaires based on *choice questions*, *Likert*, *graded questions* (in a psychometric scale), *open questions* were used.

The tools were nearly always based on original and not standardized questionnaires. Consolidated standardized tools currently used in radiology per technologies that have been consolidated for decades, such as the Picture Archive and Communication Systems [45] and the Technology Assessment Model, were not used, because they are unsuitable for unstable technologies undergoing evolution and development.

With very few exceptions, such as in [33], scholars preferred to use personal, original, and not validated/standardized questionnaires to investigate the topic. In fact, they focused on specific and new and never explored fields of the acceptance, from time to time different and not uniform (according to the felt need to produce medical knowledge), with the obvious impossibility of having specific tools ready and standardized to be reused, also considering the very recent interest in this field illustrated reported above. With very few exceptions, such as in [40,43,44], scientific societies were not involved.

4.2.2. The Tools for the Acceptance in Details

Three studies [31–33] dealt with the questionnaires on *patients* (i.e., the customer of the service/final recipient).

The first study by Fischetti et al. [31] focused on the integration of the Artificial Intelligence in the workflow. They collected opinions on several aspects of the use of Artificial Intelligence in the medical workflow from the patient entry up to the medical report.

The second study by Zhang et al. [32] proposed interviews to extract considerations on the use of the Artificial Intelligence specifically in diagnostics. The considerations were positive. The study also suggested some concerns on cybersecurity.

The third study by Ongega et al. [33] focused on the perceived perspectives on the Artificial Intelligence. The study showed: -the importance of the patients' vision of Artificial Intelligence. -The impact of the social factors. -The usefulness of the questionnaires as sensors.

The study reported by Hendrix et al. [34] focused on a first important actor (for the crucial role between the patient and the health domain): the *primary care provider*. The participants highlighted the importance of the sensitivity and other parameters in the clinical reports obtained with the Artificial Intelligence support. The use of Artificial Intelligence was considered adequate in a "triage" role to screen probable not positives without the need of the radiologist validation.

The studies reported in [35–40] investigated the opinion of other insiders, including students during the training.

The studies in [35–37] reported three investigations based on surveys submitted to *radiographers*.

In details, the study by Abuzaid et al. [35] dealt with the acceptance in the workflow. The study showed: -a generalized enthusiasm for the integration of Artificial Intelligence in the training programs. -Interest for the potential of Artificial Intelligence. -Concerns on job security. -The importance of continuous education and training.

The study by Abuzaid et al. [36] dealt with the Magnetic Resonance Imaging applications. A focus group and a questionnaire were proposed to the participants. Participants thought that Artificial Intelligence could strongly improve the workflow. In addition, in this study, the importance of the continuous education and tuned training was remarked.

The study by Giansanti et al. [37] collected opinions on the post-pandemic use of Artificial Intelligence and on the design of a structured questionnaire for the scientific societies.

The study by Abuzaid et al. [38] investigated radiologists and radiographers' opinions on the Artificial Intelligence integration into the radiology workflow. Results emphasized: -A low information on Artificial Intelligence with regards to the integration into the radiology workflow. -The importance of the design of appropriate training for both the radiographers and radiologists, with a careful consideration of the workflow.

The study by Alelyani et al. [39] investigated the acceptance in terms of attitude on radiologists, radiographers, technologists, and students. The study underlined: -The awareness of the position of Artificial Intelligence in radiology. -A higher acculturation on the Artificial Intelligence of the radiologists. -The importance of introducing specific training in the courses at the medical schools.

The study by the European Society of Radiology [40] extended the investigation on the international scene. It reported the results of a questionnaire submitted to the members of the European Society of Radiology. Questions focused on the expectations in 5–10 years. Results highlighted: -A general favorable position on Artificial Intelligence. -Detailed information on the use of Artificial Intelligence. -Opinions on the responsibility.

The study by Caparros Galan et al. [41] dealt with the opinion of the students. The participants were convinced that Artificial Intelligence could reform the radiology workflow. They did not think that this could have a dangerous impact on the work ability of radiologists. Also in this study, it was remarked the importance of the training programs on Artificial Intelligence.

The study by Di Basilio et al. [42], our companion paper (*Part 2*), proposed a questionnaire submitted to three different professionals, with different workflow backgrounds: the medical specialist, the medical physicist, and the specialist in data science. The study faced both the training and the various sectors of application of Artificial Intelligence in imaging and complementary activities. The study also highlighted the importance of the survey administration procedure, and two different methods were applied, with a different degree of interaction with the participants.

The studies in [43,44] reported two different survey administrations in this field, sponsored by two different scientific societies, and submitted on two different professionals.

The first study by Diaz et al. [43] was an international survey on medical physicists, through the related scientific society.

The second study by Coppola et al. [44] was a nationwide survey conducted on radiologists by the Italian Society of Medical and Interventional Radiology.

The first study by Diaz et al. [43] dealt with the training aspects, the involvement in Artificial Intelligence projects or activities, with the opinion on the introduction of Artificial Intelligence, and on educational interests in this field.

The second study by Coppola et al. [44] was mainly dedicated to the interaction with Artificial Intelligence (tasks by Artificial Intelligence, advantages, issues), the implications (ethical problems, risk of job loss, needs of policies), and to opinions.

5. Discussion

A Sentiment analysis review conducted on Twitter showed an increasing attention on the integration of Artificial Intelligence in Digital Radiology [46]. Other review studies clearly showed that the pandemic represented an important engine for the development of this field [47–49] and an important lesson on how to continue for the future, as highlighted in the perspective reported in [37]. Other studies considered Artificial Intelligence in Digital Radiology in terms of impact to equity [50]. There was a [50] belief that Artificial Intelligence had the strength to either widen the health inequity divide or substantially reduce it. The authors [50] believed that, with a careful attention in the use: entirely realized, Artificial Intelligence integrated in the health domain could be a part of the broader strategy convergence on local, national, and global health equity.

We fully agree with these studies [46–50]. We believe that challenges and acceptance of the integration of technology must be interconnected and go hand in hand so that expectations are not disillusioned, and we can obtain Artificial Intelligence that offers us an increasingly effective and health-oriented useful approach.

Our study in line with these considerations addressed two important points of view of the introduction of artificial intelligence in the health domain.

The first point of view related to an analysis of the challenges in the development and integration of Artificial Intelligence in the health domain.

The second point of view related to studies on the acceptance and consensus on the integration of Artificial Intelligence in the health domain mainly carried out through surveys.

5.1. The First Point of View: The Challenges

The first point of view reviewed the challenges and grouped them into six main topics. The first topic is represented by the challenges in the design and employment of the algorithms [11,12,27], in their performance improvement [11], in their potential, not also limited to the imaging field [16], and their specific application based on the solution [27]. A second topic was the revolution of the workflow [16] of the radiologist; many activities could be possible in relation to imaging and many other activities in relation to the administration of other phases of the patient management process (i.e., patient scheduling). The third topic related to the new spreading IT tools that could be strategic in the health domain [17–19]. This determined (and hence the fourth topic) the need to intensify the collaboration between [19–21] the insiders. The fifth topic is the need of targeted training also including the mobility in the territory [22,30]. The latest topic is related to the consolidation of the Artificial Intelligence system as a medical device and the related regulatory framework, from which ethics and emerging risks could not be excluded [14,24,25].

5.2. Limits and Recommendation for Future Deepening on the Challenges

Some limits and recommendation for future deepening (also because the argument was very broad and heterogeneous) emerged.

If we dwell on the algorithms, it could be seen from the study in [27] how different specific solutions based on Artificial Intelligence algorithms (suitably categorized by the authors) were necessary for different applications. In subsequent studies, it will be necessary to deepen this theme based on the categorization proposed by this study. This categorizing certainly also had an impact on IT tools and training databases [17–19,28], which could be appropriately addressed with further specific studies.

Particular attention in subsequent studies will need to be placed on the professional aspect of the radiologist and on other insiders. It will be necessary to address in detail all aspects of the change in the workflow in a specific way [16,26].

It will be essential to carry out studies on education, considering what has emerged [30], also bearing in mind the national programs. Distorting factors, cultural mediation, and the impact of training on the introduction of Artificial Intelligence will have to be investigated with also considering their relationships [15,29].

Finally, further studies will have to deepen the regulatory challenges (including also ethics) that now have been dealt with in a sectorial and patchy way [14,25].

5.3. The Second Point of View: The Tools for Investigating the Acceptance

The second point of view showed that, in the last two years, there was a notable development of studies addressing acceptance and consensus on the introduction of Artificial Intelligence in radiology using surveys [31–44]. The review showed that these studies considered different professionals (also with comparative studies between some professionals), such as radiologists, medical radiology technicians, primary care providers, students, and patients, that is, they focused on both the service providers and users, but also on subjects in training. The proposed surveys [31,32,34–44] were nearly always different and original from each other and led to very specific results.

5.4. Limits and Recommendation for Future Deepening on the Tools for Acceptance

The study revealed various limitations and the need for future developments.

First, if we look at the studies, we see that the aspects related to the opportunities and challenges have been addressed but patchy, never together and not in detail in each questionnaire. Surveys should therefore be developed that address as much as possible the aspects highlighted in the first point of view. They focused on specific, new, and never-explored fields of the acceptance, from time to time different and not uniform (according to the felt need to produce medical knowledge). In consideration of this and on the very recent interest on this topic (the first publications are from 2019), scholars used nearly always not validated surveys. Validation paths for the surveys are recommended for the future, also to allow a common language to scholars. The support of scientific societies took place in limited cases and was not always based on international initiatives [40,43]. The federations of scientific societies should be more involved to provide greater support, as highlighted in [42], since Artificial Intelligence is a crosscutting issue affecting various areas.

5.5. Limitation of the Study

The study was based on two narrative reviews dedicated to the two points of view. It analysed the scientific production in the English language as regards the publications. It did not analyse the publications in other languages (Spanish, French or Italian). The study used only two databases (PubMed and Scopus) and peer reviewed studies. Expansions of this type of survey could consider databases that include non-peer-reviewed conference articles and preprint sites. Preprint databases could give a further idea of how scholars are moving in this area by analysing articles undergoing peer review. The issue we have faced is wide-ranging and includes sub-themes that would require in-depth studies of specific studies (e.g., ethics, regulations, specificity of algorithms, just to name a few). We therefore preferred not to develop a systematic review that would have been difficult, complex and convoluted to implement, and we turned to other editorial categories admitted by the journal. Future developments could include systematic reviews targeted in the sub-themes identified.

6. Conclusions

There is great excitement around the introduction of Artificial Intelligence in the health domain and, in particular, in Digital Radiology. The pandemic seems to have given an important push towards the integration of Artificial Intelligence in Digital Radiology. It is also important that the challenges in this area be accompanied by actions in the direction of the integration of consensus conducted on insiders and citizens. The study conducted two narrative reviews, with two points of view, in parallel to take stock of both ongoing challenges and of initiatives conducted to face the acceptance and consensus in this area. The first point of view highlighted that the challenges were multifaceted and concerned various interconnected aspects. These aspects were: technological features, changes in workflows, improvement of teamwork (e.g., among data science experts and radiologists), the design of adequate training, cultural mediation actions to eliminate the factors affecting the integration, the development of adequate regulations concerning the use of Artificial Intelligence as a Medical Device in electronic health and mobile health and ethics. Survey tools based on questionnaire could be of support to monitor each of the aspects identified directly on the health domain. The second point of view showed how several studies were produced based essentially on original, non-standard, non-validated surveys, which addressed sectorial aspects on different professionals and on patients (almost always taken individually), often without the patronage of scientific societies and with local (not international) initiatives.

The study recognizes the usefulness of the questionnaire tools but suggests that they be better calibrated in order to better include all the ongoing challenges, the categories concerned, and the federations of scientific societies potentially involved. It is also desirable that future studies produce validated questionnaires that could be disseminated via international initiatives.

Author Contributions: Conceptualization, D.G.; methodology, D.G.; software, all; validation, all; formal analysis, all; investigation, all; resources, all; data curation, all; writing—original draft preparation, D.G.; writing—review and editing, D.G. and F.D.B.; visualization, all; supervision, D.G.; project administration, D.G. and F.D.B. All authors have read and agreed to the published version of the manuscript.

Funding: This research received no external funding.

Institutional Review Board Statement: Not applicable.

Informed Consent Statement: Not applicable.

Data Availability Statement: Not applicable.

Acknowledgments: The authors are thankful, with much gratitude, for the support in the qualification process: Maccioni Giovanni and Parisi Laura (Istituto Superiore di Sanità); Gianluca Esposito and Loreti Alice (Sapienza University).

Conflicts of Interest: The authors declare no conflict of interest.

References

1. Giansanti, D. The Artificial Intelligence in Digital Pathology and Digital Radiology: Where Are We? *Healthcare* **2020**, *9*, 30. [CrossRef]
2. Special Issue "The Artificial Intelligence in Digital Pathology and Digital Radiology: Where Are We?" Available online: https://www.mdpi.com/journal/healthcare/special_issues/AI_Digital_Pathology_Radiology (accessed on 23 November 2021).
3. Alsharif, M.H.; Alsharif, Y.H.; Yahya, K.; Alomari, O.A.; Albreem, M.A.; Jahid, A. Deep learning applications to combat the dissemination of COVID-19 disease: A review. *Eur. Rev. Med. Pharmacol. Sci.* **2020**, *24*, 11455–11460. [PubMed]
4. Ozsahin, I.; Sekeroglu, B.; Musa, M.S.; Mustapha, M.T.; Ozsahin, D.U. Review on Diagnosis of COVID-19 from Chest CT Images Using Artificial Intelligence. *Comput. Math. Methods Med.* **2020**, *2020*, 9756518. [CrossRef] [PubMed]
5. Luce, B.R.; Drummond, M.; Jönsson, B.; Neumann, P.J.; Schwartz, J.S.; Siebert, U.; Sullivan, S.D. EBM, HTA, and CER: Clearing the Confusion. *Milbank Q.* **2010**, *88*, 256–276. [CrossRef] [PubMed]
6. McGlynn, E.A.; Kosecoff, J.; Brook, R.H. Format and Conduct of Consensus Development Conferences. Multination Comparison. *Int. J. Technol. Assess. Health Care* **1990**, *6*, 450–469. [CrossRef]
7. Boldrini, P.; Bonaiuti, D.; Mazzoleni, S.; Posteraro, F. Rehabilitation assisted by robotic and electromechanical devices for people with neurological disabilities: Contributions for the preparation of a national conference in Italy. *Eur. J. Phys. Rehabil. Med.* **2021**, *57*, 458–459. [CrossRef]
8. Maccioni, G.; Ruscitto, S.; Gulino, R.A.; Giansanti, D. Opportunities and Problems of the Consensus Conferences in the Care Robotics. *Healthcare* **2021**, *9*, 1624. [CrossRef]
9. Evidence-Based Medicine Guidelines. Available online: https://www.ebm-guidelines.com/dtk/ebmg/home (accessed on 7 March 2022).
10. Dunnmon, J. Separating Hope from Hype: Artificial Intelligence Pitfalls and Challenges in Radiology. *Radiol. Clin. N. Am.* **2021**, *59*, 1063–1074. [CrossRef]
11. Fazal, M.I.; Patel, M.E.; Tye, J.; Gupta, Y. The past, present and future role of artificial intelligence in imaging. *Eur. J. Radiol.* **2018**, *105*, 246–250. [CrossRef]
12. Moawad, A.W.; Fuentes, D.T.; ElBanan, M.G.; Shalaby, A.S.; Guccione, J.; Kamel, S.; Jensen, C.T.; Elsayes, K.M. Artificial Intelligence in Diagnostic Radiology: Where Do We Stand, Challenges, and Opportunities. *J. Comput. Assist. Tomogr.* **2022**, *46*, 78–90. [CrossRef]
13. Kohli, M.; Alkasab, T.; Wang, K.; Heilbrun, M.E.; Flanders, A.E.; Dreyer, K.; Kahn, C.E. Bending the Artificial Intelligence Curve for Radiology: Informatics Tools From ACR and RSNA. *J. Am. Coll. Radiol.* **2019**, *16*, 1464–1470. [CrossRef] [PubMed]
14. Pesapane, F.; Volontè, C.; Codari, M.; Sardanelli, F. Artificial intelligence as a medical device in radiology: Ethical and regulatory issues in Europe and the United States. *Insights Imaging* **2018**, *9*, 745–753. [CrossRef] [PubMed]
15. Reeder, K.; Lee, H. Impact of artificial intelligence on US medical students' choice of radiology. *Clin. Imaging* **2021**, *81*, 67–71. [CrossRef] [PubMed]

16. Gampala, S.; Vankeshwaram, V.; Gadula, S.S.P. Is Artificial Intelligence the New Friend for Radiologists? A Review Article. *Cureus* **2020**, *12*, e11137. [CrossRef] [PubMed]
17. Ahmad, R. Reviewing the relationship between machines and radiology: The application of artificial intelligence. *Acta Radiol. Open* **2021**, *10*, 1–7. [CrossRef] [PubMed]
18. Hameed, B.Z.; Prerepa, G.; Patil, V.; Shekhar, P.; Raza, S.Z.; Karimi, H.; Paul, R.; Naik, N.; Modi, S.; Vigneswaran, G.; et al. Engineering and clinical use of artificial intelligence (AI) with machine learning and data science advancements: Radiology leading the way for future. *Ther. Adv. Urol.* **2021**, *13*, 17562872211044880. [CrossRef] [PubMed]
19. Kottler, N. Artificial Intelligence: A Private Practice Perspective. *J. Am. Coll. Radiol.* **2020**, *17*, 1398–1404. [CrossRef] [PubMed]
20. Martín-Noguerol, T.; Paulano-Godino, F.; López-Ortega, R.; Górriz, J.; Riascos, R.; Luna, A. Artificial intelligence in radiology: Relevance of collaborative work between radiologists and engineers for building a multidisciplinary team. *Clin. Radiol.* **2021**, *76*, 317–324. [CrossRef] [PubMed]
21. Yang, L.; Ene, I.C.; Belaghi, R.A.; Koff, D.; Stein, N.; Santaguida, P. (Lina) Stakeholders' perspectives on the future of artificial intelligence in radiology: A scoping review. *Eur. Radiol.* **2021**, *32*, 1477–1495. [CrossRef] [PubMed]
22. Pesapane, F. How scientific mobility can help current and future radiology research: A radiology trainee's perspective. *Insights Into Imaging* **2019**, *10*, 85. [CrossRef] [PubMed]
23. Pianykh, O.S.; Langs, G.; Dewey, M.; Enzmann, D.R.; Herold, C.J.; Schoenberg, S.O.; Brink, J.A. Continuous Learning AI in Radiology: Implementation Principles and Early Applications. *Radiology* **2020**, *297*, 6–14. [CrossRef]
24. D'Antonoli, T.A. Ethical considerations for artificial intelligence: An overview of the current radiology landscape. *Diagn. Interv. Radiol.* **2020**, *26*, 504–511. [CrossRef]
25. The Canadian Association of Radiologists (CAR) Artificial Intelligence Working Group; Jaremko, J.L.; Azar, M.; Bromwich, R.; Lum, A.; Cheong, L.H.A.; Gibert, M.; LaViolette, F.; Gray, B.; Reinhold, C.; et al. Canadian Association of Radiologists White Paper on Ethical and Legal Issues Related to Artificial Intelligence in Radiology. *Can. Assoc. Radiol. J.* **2019**, *70*, 107–118. [CrossRef]
26. Banja, J.; Rousselle, R.; Duszak, R., Jr.; Safdar, N.; Alessio, A.M. Sharing and Selling Images: Ethical and Regulatory Considerations for Radiologists. *J. Am. Coll. Radiol.* **2021**, *18*, 298–304. [CrossRef] [PubMed]
27. Barragán-Montero, A.; Javaid, U.; Valdés, G.; Nguyen, D.; Desbordes, P.; Macq, B.; Willems, S.; Vandewinckele, L.; Holmström, M.; Löfman, F.; et al. Artificial intelligence and machine learning for medical imaging: A technology review. *Phys. Med.* **2021**, *83*, 242–256. [CrossRef] [PubMed]
28. Cushnan, D.; Berka, R.; Bertolli, O.; Williams, P.; Schofield, D.; Joshi, I.; Favaro, A.; Halling-Brown, M.; Imreh, G.; Jefferson, E.; et al. Towards nationally curated data archives for clinical radiology image analysis at scale: Learnings from national data collection in response to a pandemic. *Digit. Health* **2021**, *7*, 1–13. [CrossRef] [PubMed]
29. Morrison, K. Artificial intelligence and the NHS: A qualitative exploration of the factors influencing adoption. *Futur. Health J.* **2021**, *8*, e648–e654. [CrossRef]
30. Fischetti, C.; Bhatter, P.; Frisch, E.; Sidhu, A.; Helmy, M.; Lungren, M.; Duhaime, E. The Evolving Importance of Artificial Intelligence and Radiology in Medical Trainee Education. *Acad. Radiol.* **2021**, *28*, 916–921. [CrossRef]
31. Lennartz, S.; Dratsch, T.; Zopfs, D.; Persigehl, T.; Maintz, D.; Hokamp, N.G.; dos Santos, D.P. Use and Control of Artificial Intelligence in Patients Across the Medical Workflow: Single-Center Questionnaire Study of Patient Perspectives. *J. Med. Int. Res.* **2021**, *23*, e24221. [CrossRef]
32. Zhang, Z.; Citardi, D.; Wang, D.; Genc, Y.; Shan, J.; Fan, X. Patients' perceptions of using artificial intelligence (AI)-based technology to comprehend radiology imaging data. *Health Inform. J.* **2021**, *27*, 1–13. [CrossRef]
33. Ongena, Y.P.; Haan, M.; Yakar, D.; Kwee, T.C. Patients' views on the implementation of artificial intelligence in radiology: Development and validation of a standardized questionnaire. *Eur. Radiol.* **2020**, *30*, 1033–1040. [CrossRef] [PubMed]
34. Hendrix, N.; Hauber, B.; Lee, C.I.; Bansal, A.; Veenstra, D.L. Artificial intelligence in breast cancer screening: Primary care provider preferences. *J. Am. Med. Inform. Assoc.* **2021**, *28*, 1117–1124. [CrossRef] [PubMed]
35. Abuzaid, M.M.; Elshami, W.; McConnell, J.; Tekin, H.O. An extensive survey of radiographers from the Middle East and India on artificial intelligence integration in radiology practice. *Health Technol.* **2021**, *11*, 1045–1050. [CrossRef]
36. Abuzaid, M.; Tekin, H.; Reza, M.; Elhag, I.; Elshami, W. Assessment of MRI technologists in acceptance and willingness to integrate artificial intelligence into practice. *Radiography* **2021**, *27*, S83–S87. [CrossRef] [PubMed]
37. Giansanti, D.; Rossi, I.; Monoscalco, L. Lessons from the COVID-19 Pandemic on the Use of Artificial Intelligence in Digital Radiology: The Submission of a Survey to Investigate the Opinion of Insiders. *Healthcare* **2021**, *9*, 331. [CrossRef]
38. Abuzaid, M.M.; Elshami, W.; Tekin, H.; Issa, B. Assessment of the Willingness of Radiologists and Radiographers to Accept the Integration of Artificial Intelligence Into Radiology Practice. *Acad. Radiol.* **2020**, *29*, 87–94. [CrossRef]
39. Alelyani, M.; Alamri, S.; Alqahtani, M.S.; Musa, A.; Almater, H.; Alqahtani, N.; Alshahrani, F.; Alelyani, S. Radiology Community Attitude in Saudi Arabia about the Applications of Artificial Intelligence in Radiology. *Healthcare* **2021**, *9*, 834. [CrossRef]
40. European Society of Radiology (ESR). Impact of artificial intelligence on radiology: A EuroAIM survey among members of the European Society of Radiology. *Insights Imaging* **2019**, *10*, 105. [CrossRef]
41. Galán, G.C.; Portero, F.S. Percepciones de estudiantes de Medicina sobre el impacto de la inteligencia artificial en radiología. *Radiología* **2021**, in press. [CrossRef]
42. Di Basilio, F.; Esposisto, G.; Monoscalco, L.; Giansanti, D. The Artificial Intelligence in Digital Radiology: Part 2: Towards an Investigation of *acceptance* and *consensus* on the Insiders. *Healthcare* **2022**, *10*, 153. [CrossRef] [PubMed]

43. Diaz, O.; Guidi, G.; Ivashchenko, O.; Colgan, N.; Zanca, F. Artificial intelligence in the medical physics community: An international survey. *Phys. Med.* **2021**, *81*, 141–146. [CrossRef] [PubMed]
44. Coppola, F.; Faggioni, L.; Regge, D.; Giovagnoni, A.; Golfieri, R.; Bibbolino, C.; Miele, V.; Neri, E.; Grassi, R. Artificial intelligence: Radiologists' expectations and opinions gleaned from a nationwide online survey. *La Radiol. Med.* **2021**, *126*, 63–71. [CrossRef] [PubMed]
45. Aldosari, B. User acceptance of a picture archiving and communication system (PACS) in a Saudi Arabian hospital radiology department. *BMC Med. Inform. Decis. Mak.* **2012**, *12*, 44. [CrossRef] [PubMed]
46. Goldberg, J.E.; Rosenkrantz, A. Artificial Intelligence and Radiology: A Social Media Perspective. *Curr. Probl. Diagn. Radiol.* **2019**, *48*, 308–311. [CrossRef] [PubMed]
47. Sideris, G.A.; Nikolakea, M.; Karanikola, A.-E.; Konstantinopoulou, S.; Giannis, D.; Modahl, L. Imaging in the COVID-19 era: Lessons learned during a pandemic. *World J. Radiol.* **2021**, *13*, 192–222. [CrossRef] [PubMed]
48. Pezzutti, D.L.; Wadhwa, V.; Makary, M.S. COVID-19 imaging: Diagnostic approaches, challenges, and evolving advances. *World J. Radiol.* **2021**, *13*, 171–191. [CrossRef] [PubMed]
49. El Naqa, I.M.; Li, H.; Fuhrman, J.D.; Hu, Q.; Gorre, N.; Chen, W.; Giger, M.L. Lessons learned in transitioning to AI in the medical imaging of COVID-19. *J. Med. Imaging* **2021**, *8* (Suppl. S1), 010902. [CrossRef]
50. Currie, G.; Rohren, E. Social Asymmetry, Artificial Intelligence and the Medical Imaging Landscape. *Semin. Nucl. Med.* **2021**, *in press*. [CrossRef] [PubMed]

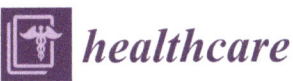

Article

The Artificial Intelligence in Digital Radiology: *Part 2*: Towards an Investigation of *acceptance* and *consensus* on the Insiders

Francesco Di Basilio [1], Gianluca Esposisto [1], Lisa Monoscalco [2] and Daniele Giansanti [3],*

[1] Facoltà di Medicina e Psicologia, Sapienza University, Piazzale Aldo Moro, 00185 Rome, Italy; fdibasilio@hotmail.com (F.D.B.); gianluca.esposito.sapienza@gmail.com (G.E.)
[2] Faculty of Engineering, Tor Vergata University, 00133 Rome, Italy; lisamonoscalco@hotmail.com
[3] Centre Tisp, Istituto Superiore di Sanità, 00161 Rome, Italy
* Correspondence: daniele.giansanti@iss.it; Tel.: +39-06-49902701

Abstract: *Background.* The study deals with the introduction of the artificial intelligence in digital radiology. There is a growing interest in this area of scientific research in *acceptance* and *consensus* studies involving both insiders and the public, based on surveys focused mainly on single professionals. *Purpose.* The goal of the study is to perform a contemporary investigation on the *acceptance* and the *consensus* of the three key professional figures approaching in this field of application: (1) Medical specialists in image diagnostics: the medical specialists (MS)s; (2) experts in physical imaging processes: the medical physicists (MP)s; (3) AI designers: specialists of applied sciences (SAS)s. *Methods.* Participants (MSs = 92: 48 males/44 females, averaged age 37.9; MPs = 91: 43 males/48 females, averaged age 36.1; SAS = 90: 47 males/43 females, averaged age 37.3) were properly recruited based on specific training. An electronic survey was designed and submitted to the participants with a wide range questions starting from the training and background up to the different applications of the AI and the environment of application. *Results.* The results show that generally, the three professionals show (a) a high degree of encouraging agreement on the introduction of AI both in imaging and in non-imaging applications using both standalone applications and/or *mHealth/eHealth*, and (b) a different consent on AI use depending on the training background. *Conclusions.* The study highlights the usefulness of focusing on both the three key professionals and the usefulness of the investigation schemes facing a wide range of issues. The study also suggests the importance of different methods of administration to improve the adhesion and the need to continue these investigations both with federated and specific initiatives.

Keywords: e-health; medical devices; m-health; digital-radiology; picture archive and communication system; artificial-intelligence; electronic surveys; chest CT; chest radiography; acceptance; consensus

Citation: Di Basilio, F.; Esposisto, G.; Monoscalco, L.; Giansanti, D. The Artificial Intelligence in Digital Radiology: *Part 2*: Towards an Investigation of *acceptance* and *consensus* on the Insiders. *Healthcare* **2022**, *10*, 153. https://doi.org/10.3390/healthcare10010153

Academic Editor: Norbert Hosten

Received: 9 November 2021
Accepted: 10 January 2022
Published: 14 January 2022

Publisher's Note: MDPI stays neutral with regard to jurisdictional claims in published maps and institutional affiliations.

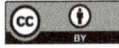

Copyright: © 2022 by the authors. Licensee MDPI, Basel, Switzerland. This article is an open access article distributed under the terms and conditions of the Creative Commons Attribution (CC BY) license (https://creativecommons.org/licenses/by/4.0/).

1. Introduction

Artificial Intelligence and Digital Radiology

The standardization of digital radiology caused important changes in the field of organ and functional diagnostics. This regards both the diagnostics and the interventional radiology [1,2]. It has led to exceptional changes in the organization of work and reporting processes. Furthermore, it pushed the digitization and computerization [3,4]. This solved and simplified many organizational problems, such as the organization of the archives, even if new ones appeared, such as those related to cybersecurity [5,6]. Today, digital radiology (DR) embraces a wide sector of diagnostic scenarios, also including sectors not directly related with the ionizing radiation, such as magnetic resonance and echography [7–9]. Those imaging sectors using DICOM are united under the hat of digital radiology [10–13]. Now, we are facing the possible impact of research on the health domain [14]. An important engine in this context is represented by the research efforts during the COVID-19 pandemic. For example, research on chest CT/radiography has opened important discussions and scenarios [15–18].

AI, a field of computer science [19], when used in the *health domain* is considered a tool able to perform tasks normally requiring human intelligence [20–23] that in recent years have been applied in various health-related areas, such as cancer detection [24], dementia classification [25], and drug design [26], to name a few.

If we consider the potential of AI in DR, the applications are multiple.

We need to consider four important *points of view* when we enter the field of DR [27,28]:

1. A *first point* of view is that DR includes different imaging sectors where it can potentially be applied. If we exclude imaging processes that do not involve ionizing radiation, we can identify the following sectors, both with reference to organ and total body diagnostics:
   a. Interventional radiology
   b. Diagnostic radiology (radiology, CT)
   c. Nuclear magnetic resonance
   d. Positron emission tomography
   e. amma chamber

2. A *second point of view* is represented by the transversal sectors that embrace these disciplines in which AI can play an important role:
   a. Therapy
   b. Prevention
   c. Quality control
   d. Risk assessment

3. A *third point of view* is represented by the AI app distribution methods. In fact, we must not forget that AI, in the context of DR, has a future of standardization related to software for medical devices [29]. This software has different implications if it is used *standalone* or on the network, and if it is networked through *eHealth* or *mHealth* solutions. The implications also concern important aspects of cybersecurity [30].

4. A *fourth point of view* is represented by the specific training that must include AI and also the related disciplines such as informatics, medical imaging and the technologies for biomedical app.

The passage of the AI into the routine of the DR (including the above listed *points of view*) must take place through an approach that provides for the transfer of evidence-based medicine (EBM) to the operational processes of the *health domain*, using all the available agreement tools, which include guidelines [31], technology assessment (TA) such as HTA and CER [32], and consensus conferences [33]. The latest definition of EBM, by Eddy [34], also considers the development of evidence-based policies in a multi-dimensional space of the *health domain*, involving quality, acceptance, consensus, and cost-effectiveness analysis. All the agreement tools will therefore also be based, as in other disciplines, on the *acceptance and consensus* of both the insiders and the public who will help to express important positions. A PubMed search in this area with the two keys [35,36]:

(acceptance) AND (artificial intelligence [Title/Abstract]) AND Radiology)

(consensus) AND (artificial intelligence [Title/Abstract]) AND Radiology)

shows (Figure 1) 83 results, of which 77 from 2019 to today for the acceptance and 23 results for the consensus, all comprised from 2019 to today.

This means that acceptance and consensus have become a priority on this issue over the past two years. Among the emerging tools in this area, we find the surveys useful as sensors for stakeholders and managers in general. These surveys [37–47] focused on some of the actors that revolve around this area: radiologists, radiographers, primary care providers (PCP), students, and patients, that is, both on service providers and users, but also on subjects in training. The studies on patients [37–39] have highlighted the curiosity and non-opposition to these techniques, together with the need to create culture, the need to educate on the issue and the fear for the aspects of cybersecurity in integration with *eHealth* and *mHealth*. The students [47] showed curiosity and optimism but complained about a lack of adequate training and the need to integrate specific modules into the training programs. Openings towards these solutions have emerged from studies on *radiologists* and *radiographers* [41–46] accompanied by the strong desire to have an important role in future *work-flow* modification processes and adequate training. In almost all studies, with rare exceptions such as [39], free and non-standardized questionnaires were used through validation processes, indicating that scholars, at this historical moment, are relying on their creativity to create increasingly innovative and adaptive questionnaires. Instruments, such as the TAM, widely used in radiology were not used [48].

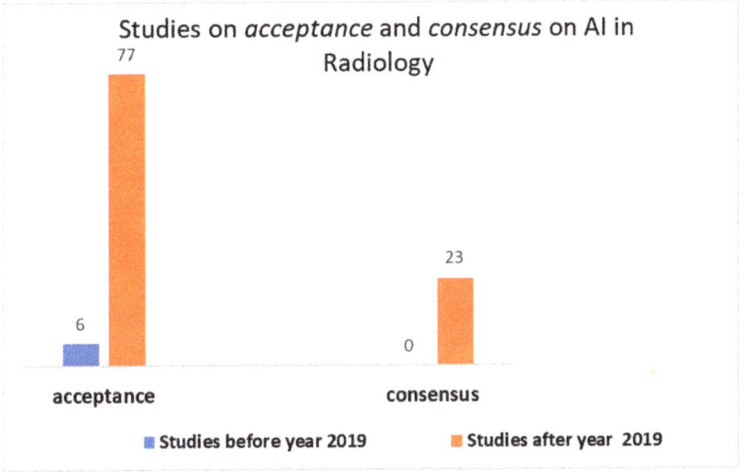

Figure 1. Output of the search on PubMed on acceptance and consensus on AI in radiology.

What emerges from these studies are the following *needs of deepening* for further study in the surveys. Many figures have been thought of, such as the PCP [40], but others have been neglected. No studies have been identified on the specialists of applied sciences of artificial intelligence systems. In rare cases, surveys have been carried out which involved several professional figures, such as in [44,45], which involved both *radiologists* and *radiographers*. Our hypothesis is that the AI acceptance survey in radiology:

- must consider the above-listed (1–4) points of views, not limited to imaging and including the integration into *eHealth* and *mHealth* [49];
- must consider all the *involved professionals who have different training and a different work-flow and therefore different expectations from AI.*

Some studies on the design and test of AI solutions are clearly highlighting the importance of the team [50]. This team comprehends *(with a natural osmosis of skills)*:

- the medical physics;
- the medical specialist;
- the specialist in applied sciences.

A preparatory and preliminary step to the introduction of the AI in the clinical practice should directly face the *consensus/acceptance*. It emerges, based on the above, that important actors are undoubtedly (Figure 2): *medical specialists (MS)s, medical physicists (MP)s,* and *specialists of applied sciences (SAS)s*. MSs are a strategic role in the decision flow. MPs control the physical process. SASs design and maintain the AI tools (such as the biomedical engineers and technicians/technologists of radiology). The purpose of the study was: (a) to focus on these three professionals to investigate their *acceptance and consensus*; (b) to design and submit them a properly electronic survey for the investigation, with a wide range of features considering the highlighted needs of deepening the points listed above.

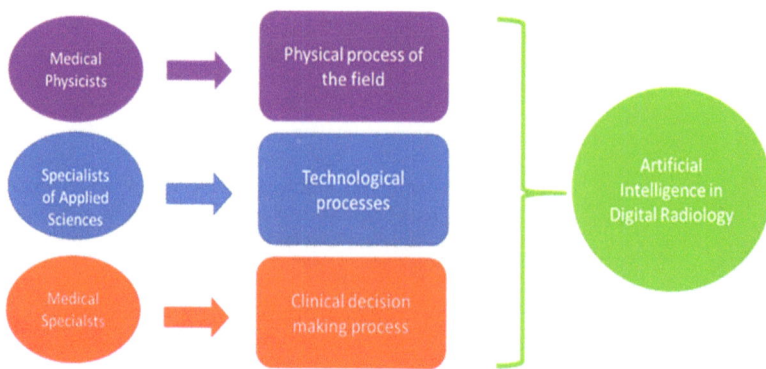

Figure 2. Interconnection among experts and AI.

2. Methods

In line with the aim of the study, we decided to develop a survey.

The methodology comprehended: (I) the choice of the tool for the design of the electronic survey and (II) the adequacy to regulations; (III) the design of the survey based on the chosen tool respecting the wide range features to investigate; (IV) the dissemination on a population; (V) the data analysis based on an effective statistical approach. The questionnaire was developed using Microsoft Forms. It adhered to the SURGE Checklist [51] for the development and administration of the survey. The statistics followed two steps:

- Verification of data normality;
- Application of the ANOVA with a P lower than 0.01 for the significance of differences.

For the statistical confidence interval, we set a goal of 95%.

We considered that, among the most used tests to verify the normality, there are: (a) the Shapiro–Wilk test, which is preferable for a small sample; (b) the Kolmogorov–Smirnov test, which is instead used for more numerous samples. The samples in this study are small; therefore, we used the normality test of Shapiro–Wilk. We focused on the key figures (Figure 2) for the investigation.

The electronic survey was designed to face a wide range of features (starting from the training and the background, up to the application of the AI and the environment of application) using: *choice questions, open questions, graded questions, and Likert* (Figure 3).

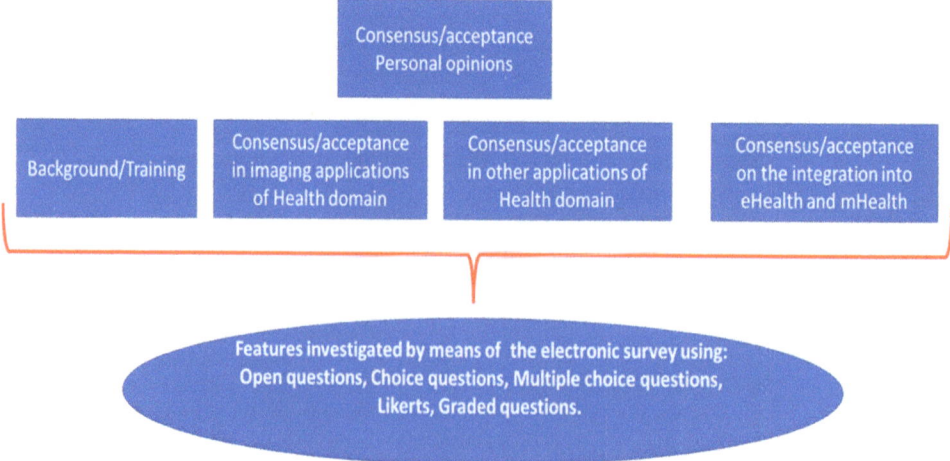

Figure 3. Features investigated by means of the electronic survey.

Both in the graded questions and in the Likert questions we fixed a six-level psychometric scale; it was therefore possible to assign a minimum score of one and a maximum score of six with a theoretical mean value (*TMV*) of 3.5. The *TMV* can be referred to for comparison in the analysis of the answers. An average value of the answers below TMV indicates a more negative than positive response. An average value above *TMV* indicates a more positive than negative response. The survey was accompanied by a brief description of the topic that would be addressed, clearly illustrating that the focus was related to the introduction of AI in digital radiology.

For the recruitment, we considered the three figures as planned, who, we remember, are medical specialists (MS), medical physicists (MP), specialists of applied sciences (SAS). All figures have a different role with AI in DR; this implies a different vision/opinion/consensus. The recruitment of these figures was very complex given that they belong to very different sectors, to different scientific societies. Currently, in Italy, there are 334 scientific societies [52]. We followed two paths that we have traced:

First way

In Italy, there are also federations of scientific societies that favor a scientific osmosis between the various scientific societies.

As regards the three professionals, we referred to:

- FEDERATION OF ITALIAN MEDICAL-SCIENTIFIC SOCIETIES [53] (includes associations such as the Italian association of medical and health physics and other relevant scientific societies and other societies operating in the Medical Diagnostics and in related fields) mainly for the first two professionals MPs and MSs but also for the SASs.
- FEDERATION OF SCIENTIFIC AND TECHNICAL ASSOCIATIONS [54] (contains the National Group of Bioengineering and other relevant scientific societies) and FEDERATION OF SCIENTIFIC ASSOCIATIONS OF RADIOLOGY TECHNICIANS [55] (contains for example the Italian association of system administrators and telemedicine, association of interventional radiology technicians, Health Imaging Sciences Association, and other relevant societies) mainly for the SASs but also for the other professionals.

It was possible for us to have lists of congresses in which to collect preliminary adhesions of interest for the project, in the presence, with contacts, encounters, discussions. A WhatsApp group was created to which the invitation and the anonymous questionnaire were sent, with a brief description and a recall of the discussion. In this way, it was possible to send the survey anonymously.

Second way

Sending was also carried out through our networks of WhatsApp, also following a peer-to-peer mechanism.

Table 1 reports the participants, the participants agreeing to continue after opening the questionnaire, and the related demographic characteristics. The average age of those who filled out the survey was not high. This depends on the very innovative and recent typology of the proposed theme, which was more attractive and inclusive (due to the training received) for the younger population.

Table 1. Characteristics of the participants in the study and the final involvement.

	Participants	Participants Agreeing to Continue/Passing the Requirement	Males/Females	Min Age/Max Age	Mean Age
MSs	111	108/92	48/44	32/43	37.9
MPs	105	97/91	43/48	31/41	36.1
SASs	99	93/90	47/43	33/40	37.3

Figures A1 and A2 in the Appendix A show a sample of the questionnaire. It was converted from the Italian language into the English language.

3. Results

3.1. Outcome of the Closed Questions from the Survey

The eS contained a specific question relating to an adequate level of knowledge on AI to participate (through the attendance, for example, of specific academic and/or post-academic training). Only those who passed this requirement were admitted to the study. The results are organized into five tables. The first table (Table 2) concerns the *training on AI* aspects.

Table 2. Specific outcome of the *perceived training*.

Knowledge	MSs Score	MPs Score	SASs Score	ANOVA p
AI (general)	4.56	4.38	4.51	$p > 0.1$
AI (informatics)	4.33	4.24	5.22	$p < 0.01$
AI (medical imaging)	4.98	5.07	5.02	$p > 0.1$
Technologies for biomedical Apps	4.32	5.03	5.11	$p < 0.01$

The second table (Table 3) concerns the consent/opinion on the application of AI specifically related to *medical imaging*.

Table 3. Specific outcome of the opinion on the application *on the medical imaging*.

Application of AI in:	MSs Score	MPs Score	SASs Score	ANOVA p
	4.26	4.18	4.11	$p > 0.1$
Interventional radiology	4.54	4.39	4.41	$p > 0.1$
Diagnostic radiology (radiology, CT, etc.)	4.26	4.28	4.31	$p > 0.1$
Nuclear magnetic resonance	4.61	4.69	4.72	$p > 0.1$
Positron emission tomography	4.53	4.38	4.52	$p > 0.1$
Gamma chamber	4.44	4.39	4.43	$p > 0.1$

The third table (Table 4) concerns the consent/opinion on the application on other medical aspects not directly related to medical imaging (*therapy, risk analysis, quality control, prevention*).

Table 4. Specific outcome of the opinion on the application of AI different from imaging.

Application of AI (Non Imaging)	MSs Score	MPs Score	SASs Score	ANOVA p
Risk assessment	4.82	4.21	4.13	$p < 0.01$
Therapy	5.21	4.65	4.52	$p < 0.01$
Prevention	5.11	4.02	4.11	$p < 0.01$
Quality Control	4.12	5.07	5.12	$p < 0.01$

The fourth table (Table 5) concerns aspects on how it is considered convenient to approach AI regarding the information available (*eHealth, mHealth, Standalone*, both *eHealth* and *mHealth*) [43].

Table 5. Specific outcome of the opinion on the use/delivery of the AI.

Scheme	MSs Score	MPs Score	SASs Score	ANOVA p
eHealth	4.72	4.66	3.93	$p < 0.01$
mHealth	4.55	4.62	3.89	$p < 0.01$
Both eHealth and mHealth	4.58	4.62	3.86	$p < 0.01$
Standalone	5.33	5,24	5.17	$p > 0.1$

Table 6 reports the output on a graded question related on the generalized optimism related to the general use of AI.

Table 6. Optimism on the AI use.

Optimism	MSs Score	MPs Score	SASs Score	ANOVA p
AI (All)	4.58	4.57	4.53	$p > 0.1$
AI (people dealing with AI in the workplace)	4.98	4.96	4.93	$p > 0.1$

Data were successfully preliminarily tested for the normality using the Shapiro test.

With regards to the *training* (Table 2), the subjects passing the barrier showed a high degree (score > TMV) in the three groups. However, the behavior was different in some cases. The ANOVA test highlighted some differences dependent on the different background: (a) in the case of *informatics*, where the SAS recorded a higher score; (b) in the case of *technologies for biomedical apps*, where both MPs and SASs showed a higher score.

We also included open-ended questions to investigate whether participants had direct experience (i.e., *training on the job*) in AI applied to the clinic. As far as MS is concerned, this can be represented, for example, by a direct experience of the clinical decision supported by AI. As for the MPs and SAS, this can be represented by direct activity on equipment equipped with AI systems as regards activities that can go from development to calibration and/or quality control. From these open questions, after classification and categorization, we found that a small percentage of respondents said they had or have such direct experience. A total of 14.3% of the MSs, 13.9% of the MPs, and 14.8% of the SASs had direct experience *of training on the job*. The *trained on the job* individuals showed a higher value of general optimism in the use of AI, uniform for the three groups (Table 6). With regards to the applications in medical imaging (Table 3), the subjects passing the barrier showed a high degree (score > TMV) in the three groups. The behavior was uniform. The ANOVA test highlighted no differences in all the issues among the groups. It is here evident that even if the background is different—*the MSs faced the diagnostic more; the MPS faced the imaging processes more; the SASs faced the technologies more*—the diversity compensated among themselves.

With regards to the use of AI in applications in the general fields (excluding the medical imaging) (Table 4), the subjects passing the barrier showed a high degree (score > TMV) in the three groups. However, the behavior was different in some cases. The ANOVA test highlighted some differences, dependent on the different background: (a) in the case of the more medical issues, *risk assessment*, *therapy*, and *prevention* where the MSs recorded a higher score; (b) in the case of *quality control*, both the MPs and SAS showed a higher score in this issue that is most related to the specific background. The opinion on the way of using/providing the AI (Table 5) is reported in consideration of the importance of the integration into the *eHealth* and *mHealth* [49]. With regards to this issue, the subjects passing the barrier showed a high degree (score > TMV) in the three groups, with a preference for the standalone approach. The preference for the standalone is probably due to the awareness on the exposition to the cyber risk. However, the behavior was different in some cases, where the SAS showed a lower score for the issues *mHealth*, *eHealth*, and *both*. This relates to the higher training in *informatics* (see above) that leads to higher awareness on the cyber risks when not applying AI in standalone.

3.2. Key Considerations from the Submission Process and Suggestions from the Open Questions

3.2.1. Adhesion to the Survey

This type of administration will be more and more widespread in the future. Analyzing the peculiarities and the outcome of the recruitment mechanisms is therefore of primary importance. The two administrations took place in different time intervals to allow the evaluation of the contributions to the total data collection. Two paths were followed in our study. The first one began in 2019 with the collection of availability in presence at congresses with the possibility of an oral interaction/discussion and subsequent sending with WhatsApp.

The second was without oral discussion and was based on peer-to-peer sending via WhatsApp. Figure 4 highlights how the greatest contribution to data collection came through the first method based on (traditional) oral communication. Figure 5 shows the percentages of adhesions with respect to each method. The results show that the first method had a surprisingly higher percentage of adhesion. This demonstrates how the oral communication made of the three verbal, para-verbal, and non-verbal components continues to maintain a greater grip than a communication made with chat only.

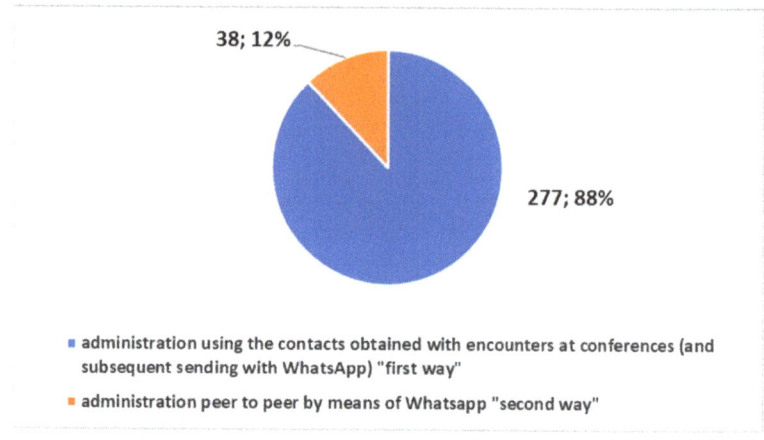

Figure 4. Contributions to the survey by the two different methods.

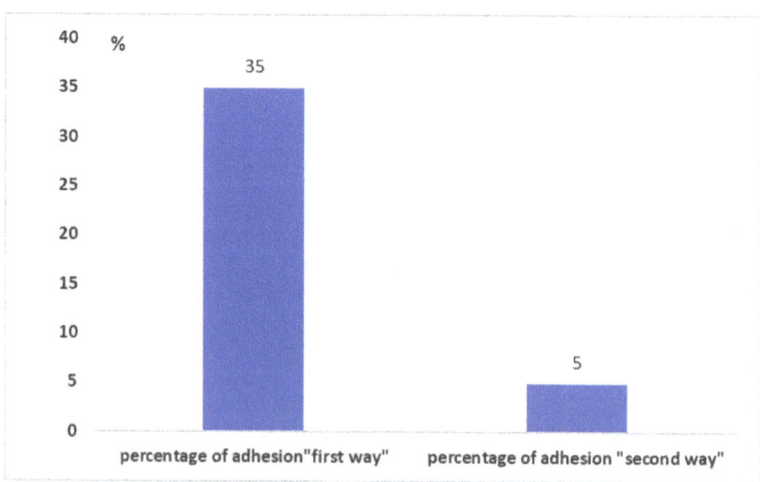

Figure 5. The percentage of adhesion to the survey by the two different methods.

3.2.2. Outcome from the Open Question

In the survey to question No. 13, we optionally offered the possibility of reporting comments and observations.

Twenty-one interviewed people reported an observation or comment. We analyzed the comments that highlighted critical issues and suggestions for improvement, and we carried out datamining, which was followed by categorization.

Figure 6 reports the following points as important suggestions for improvement based on the order of the frequency of occurrence:

o to request the CV in a subsection with a series of targeted questions;
o to prepare a survey for each type of professional;
o to refine the survey within scientific societies;
o to offer a question/answer grid with very specific training aspects of AI.

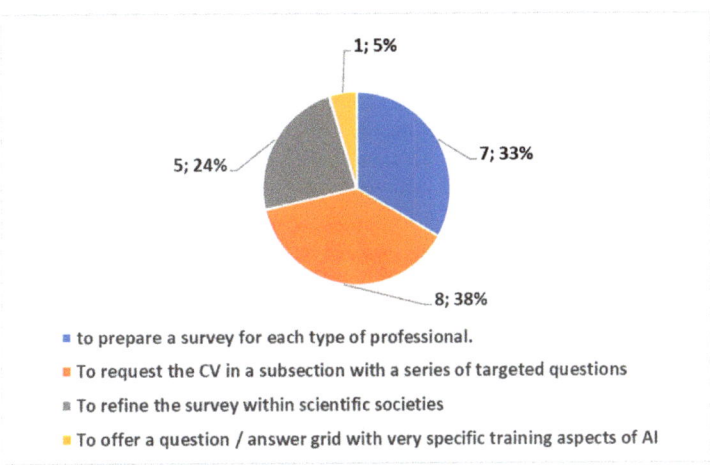

Figure 6. Suggestions for improvement with the obtained frequency of occurrence.

4. Discussion

We are undoubtedly about to face another important change in the world of digital radiology [14]: the introduction of AI in clinical practice. During the pandemic, the importance and potential of AI clearly emerged in two sectors of digital radiology: chest CT and chest radiography [15–18,43]. However, even before the pandemic, we were already talking about this phenomenon affecting the *health domain*, especially the sectors where the conversion to *digital health* has been heavy, such as the DR [27,28], thanks to the DICOM standardization process. DICOM is the container of the information arranged into pixels and/or voxels after the process of image acquisition. The pixels and/or voxels used as AI input carry different information of the investigated biomedical target. The information in those elements is related to the *physical process* (X-rays, gamma rays, magnetic fields, ultrasounds, etc.). Three elements play an important role: (1) the *physical process (PP)*, which depends on the physical fields used (X-rays, magnetic field, ultrasound, etc.); (2) the *technological process (TP)*, which concerns both the technologies for capturing information starting from the physical process, and the software implementation of AI-based algorithms; (3) the *decision-making process (DP)*, which must consider the outcome from the TP based on a PP and the human decision based on *medical knowledge* functionally related to both the TP and PP.

It is for this reason that it is important that the experts of the DP, TP, and PP work are connected in the process of AI introduction and in the related investigations.

It should also be borne in mind that in addition to diagnostic imaging, other AI applications used for *categorization into non-imaging* problems [9,27] (non-imaging categorization) were considered in the study. These range from risk analysis up to quality control. We also found it important to consider in the study how AI is delivered, whether it is delivered in standalone mode, or based on *mHealth* or *eHealth* [49]. In light of what has been illustrated above, we have decided to consider in the study the three figures of MSs, MPs, and SASs connected to (1,2) to investigate the *consensus and acceptance* by means of an eS. From a general point of view, these three professional figures showed a high degree of acceptance of the introduction of AI both in imaging and in non-imaging applications, using both standalone and network modes (*mHealth* or *eHealth*). Specifically, through a statistical assessment based on ANOVA, we were able to see a different way of approaching AI. This approach was uniform when considering AI applied to imaging. The approach was not uniform when considering the non-imaging applications and the delivery methods. Subjects with a background comprehending direct training on the job focused on AI showed the highest optimism. From a general point of view, the study highlights the usefulness of investigating the inclusion of AI through an eS, the usefulness of doing so based on three categories of experts (MSs; MPs; SASs), and the general optimism in the introduction of AI in digital radiology.

The background plays an important role in relation to the approach to AI. In the scientific literature, various studies already involved radiologists (key figures in the clinical decision) to perform reader studies. In a certain sense, if we look at the study proposed on a direct application of AI [50] in its entirety, we realize that regarding the enhancement of AI, the study we have proposed is in a complementary position. Our study directly focuses to the three involved professionals, having an active role in the flow from the tool design up to the decision [50]. Our study is in line with the studies based on surveys [37–47]; the submission of original surveys allows to obtain strategic information. In addition to similar studies, our study addressed the innovation of submitting the same survey to three key figures operating in the TP, PP, and DP. Furthermore, considering the needs that emerged from previous studies, our study proposed different survey schemes based on Likert/graded questions at six psychometric levels to have different quantitative outcomes, useful for categorizations.

A first scheme dealt with the educational, academic, and post-academic training aspects on modules relevant to the knowledge bases useful in this field.

A second scheme addressed the imaging aspects in detail, focusing on the different compatible DICOM tools used in DR.

The third scheme addressed the aspects of AI external to imaging but always relevant to the *work flow* (quality control, risk assessment, therapy and prevention) [27,28].

A fourth scheme was dedicated to integration with *eHealth and mHealth* [49], strategic for addressing important aspects such as cybersecurity.

From a general point of view, the study differs from other initiatives in this direction [56–59]. Furthermore, it offers to the scholars a complementary contribution and therefore complementary results if compared to study based on surveys [58,59]. Our proposed survey (see Appendix A) comprehends 13 questions (23 if we consider that the Likert has submodules): (a) it is oriented to all three professions potentially involved, (b) it goes into detail in the application of AI in the different sectors of imaging with a specific Likert and by means of another Likert in the application of AI in the translational sectors of the *health domain*, and (c) it addresses aspects of network integration (standalone, mHealth, eHealth) important for the impact on software medical device and cybersecurity. We have used several modules detailing the *choice questions, the open questions, the open large questions, and two modules used to give a psycho/sociometric assessment* (now currently used in the life sciences): the *graded questions and the Likert*. In addition, in our survey, there was also the possibility of supplementing the demographic information (including training) and work activity with two specific open questions, one *open large question* dedicated to the insertion of the CV, and one *open question* dedicated to the description of one's own working activity.

The two surveys in [58,59] are in turn complementary; they are each dedicated to a specific professional figure and with different focuses.

The survey reported in [58] concerns a national audience, is focused on the MSs, and is made up of 13 questions: 4 dedicated to demographic aspects (age, region, activity, position and job site), 3 dedicated to interaction with AI (tasks by AI, advantages, issues), 3 dedicated to implications (ethical problems, risk of job loss, needs of policies), and other questions in complement, such as the opinion on the definition of AI.

The other survey [59] concerns an international audience, is dedicated to the figure of the MP, and consists of 25 questions. The first eight deal with the training aspects, the involvement in AI projects and with the activities and the opinion on the introduction of AI. Questions 9 to 17 all concern the collection of educational interests in a specific way and the opinions on the integration of the CV in future activities. An open question (number 18) is free. The final questions are all focused on demographics.

Our survey was submitted through two channels, both electronic (one of which, however, was also based on a preliminary in-person presentation of the initiative), which were evaluated. Part of the analysis was dedicated to the observations and criticalities that emerged, as well as specifically collected.

Both the surveys reported in [58,59] were administered with purely electronic methods, and there was no comparison between different modalities. They did not use graded questions and Likert questions. Furthermore, the critical issues to be addressed to improve these initiatives were not collected from both the surveys.

As regards the dissemination of the survey, our study shows that a preliminary contact in presence (followed by an electronic transmission) improves the participation rate. This suggests for the future to address these initiatives by preceding them by preliminary face-to-face meetings (for example, in focus groups or congresses). Regarding suggestions for improvement and development, it should be noted that those proposals that have had a frequency greater than 1 push towards a structured request in a grid of the CV, a specialization of the survey for the different professionals, and a refinement in scientific societies.

Considering these observations and what has emerged, the continuation of these initiatives in both a specialized and federated way is certainly desirable. It is hoped that the AI will be an opportunity to give birth to scientific federations that allow for in-depth initiatives in both a specific and confederate way.

5. Conclusions

The introduction of AI into clinical practice is now an unstoppable process that will take this discipline from research to routine use. Many professionals from now to the future will be involved, and it will be necessary to provide for targeted consensus actions to issue appropriate recommendations. Guidelines, TA reports, and consensus conferences, spread by scientific societies in the sector, for example, will in the future also use approaches based on surveys that scholars are currently developing.

Initiatives aimed at creating position papers in this area will be more and more frequent and will involve more and more teams of professionals, as in [56], where *medical physics* and *radiologists* have worked. Both national [57,58] and international [59] scientific societies could play an important role in the improvement and dissemination of these surveys, which could play a strategic role in monitoring the topic. It will also be important that scientific societies representing the different actors work as a team in initiatives that could possibly lead to stable and standardized international monitoring actions.

Author Contributions: Conceptualization, D.G.; methodology, D.G. and F.D.B.; software, D.G. and L.M.; validation, D.G., G.E. and F.D.B.; formal analysis, All; investigation, All; resources, not applicable; data curation, D.G. and L.M.; writing—original draft preparation, D.G.; writing—review and editing, All; visualization, All; supervision, D.G.; project administration, D.G. and L.M.; funding acquisition, not applicable. All authors have read and agreed to the published version of the manuscript.

Funding: This research received no external funding.

Institutional Review Board Statement: Not applicable.

Informed Consent Statement: Not applicable.

Data Availability Statement: Not applicable.

Conflicts of Interest: The authors declare no conflict of interest.

Abbreviations

Acronym	Description
AI	Artificial intelligence
CT	Computerized tomography
MP	Medical physicist
SAS	Specialists of applied sciences
MS	Medical specialist
DICOM	Digital imaging and communications in medicine
DR	Digital radiology
TA	Technology assessment
HTA	Health technology assessment
CER	Comparative effectiveness research
PCP	Primary care provider
TP	Technological process
TMV	Theorical mean value
PP	Physical process
DP	Decision-making process
ANOVA	Analysis of variance
eHealth	Electronic health
mHealth	Mobile health

Appendix A

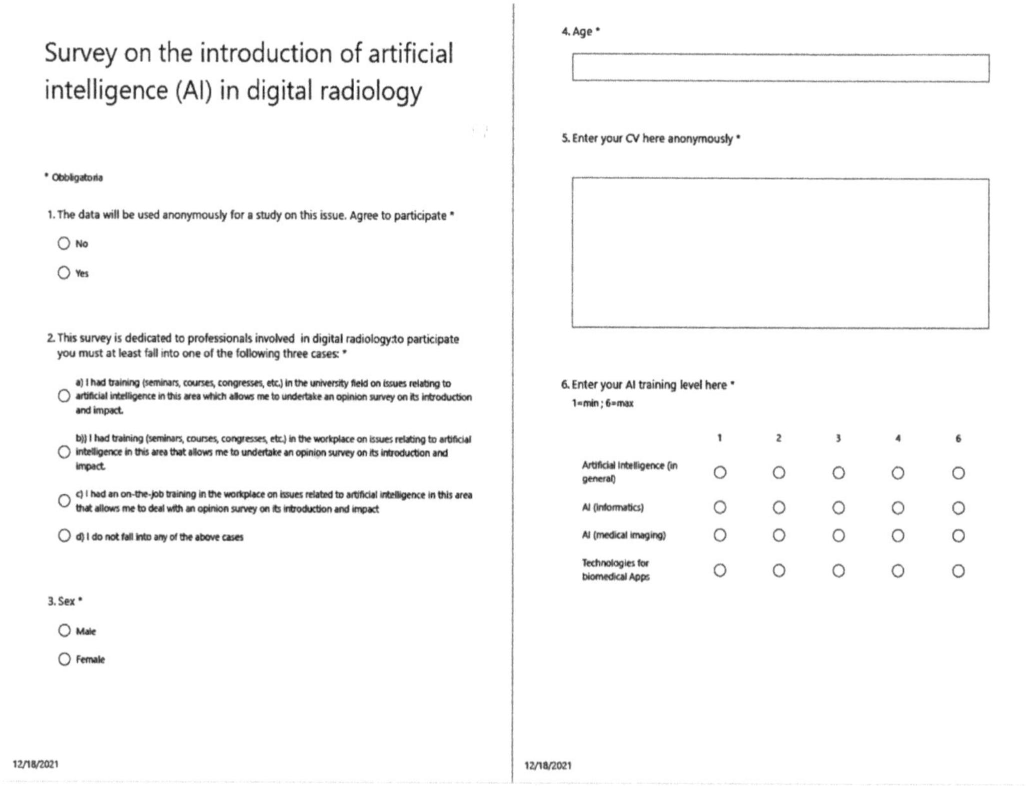

Survey on the introduction of artificial intelligence (AI) in digital radiology

* Obbligatoria

1. The data will be used anonymously for a study on this issue. Agree to participate *

○ No

○ Yes

2. This survey is dedicated to professionals involved in digital radiology:to participate you must at least fall into one of the following three cases: *

○ a) I had training (seminars, courses, congresses, etc.) in the university field on issues relating to artificial intelligence in this area which allows me to undertake an opinion survey on its introduction and impact.

○ b)) I had training (seminars, courses, congresses, etc.) in the workplace on issues relating to artificial intelligence in this area that allows me to undertake an opinion survey on its introduction and impact.

○ c) I had an on-the-job training in the workplace on issues related to artificial intelligence in this area that allows me to deal with an opinion survey on its introduction and impact

○ d) I do not fall into any of the above cases

3. Sex *

○ Male

○ Female

12/18/2021

4. Age *

5. Enter your CV here anonymously *

6. Enter your AI training level here *
1=min ; 6=max

	1	2	3	4	6
Artificial Intelligence (in general)	○	○	○	○	○
AI (informatics)	○	○	○	○	○
AI (medical imaging)	○	○	○	○	○
Technologies for biomedical Apps	○	○	○	○	○

12/18/2021

Figure A1. An example of the survey (first print screen).

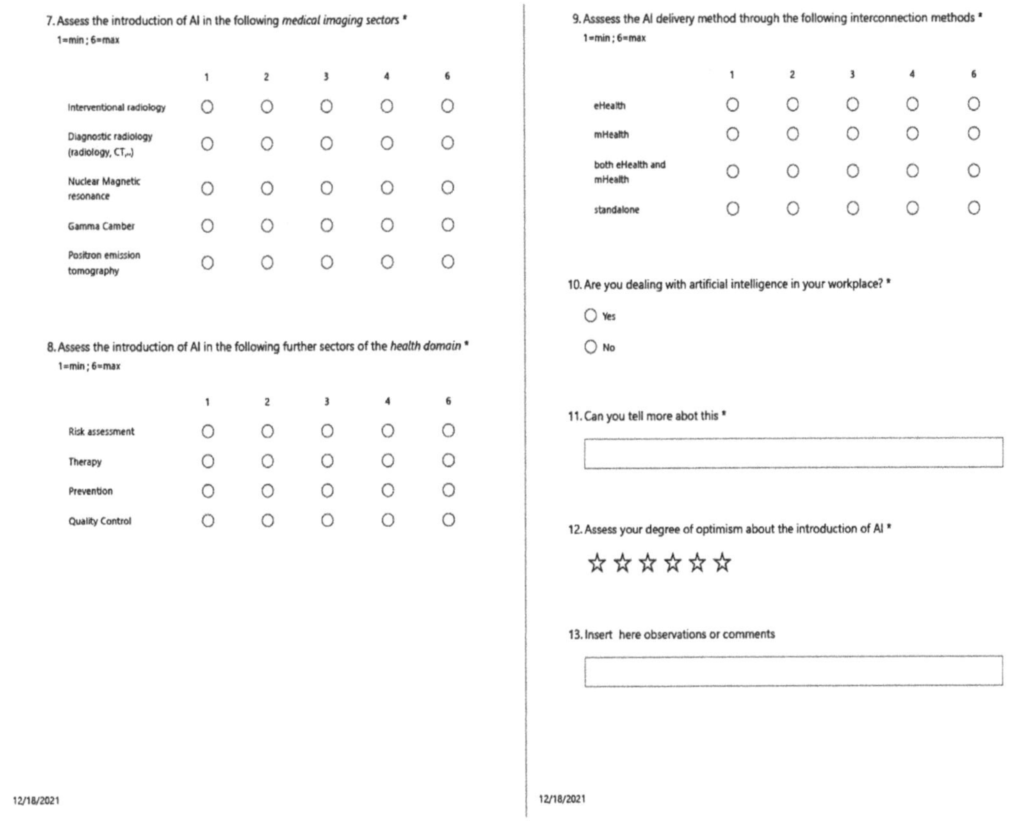

7. Assess the introduction of AI in the following *medical imaging sectors* *
1=min ; 6=max

	1	2	3	4	6
Interventional radiology	O	O	O	O	O
Diagnostic radiology (radiology, CT,..)	O	O	O	O	O
Nuclear Magnetic resonance	O	O	O	O	O
Gamma Camber	O	O	O	O	O
Positron emission tomography	O	O	O	O	O

8. Assess the introduction of AI in the following further sectors of the *health domain* *
1=min ; 6=max

	1	2	3	4	6
Risk assessment	O	O	O	O	O
Therapy	O	O	O	O	O
Prevention	O	O	O	O	O
Quality Control	O	O	O	O	O

12/18/2021

9. Asssess the AI delivery method through the following interconnection methods *
1=min ; 6=max

	1	2	3	4	6
eHealth	O	O	O	O	O
mHealth	O	O	O	O	O
both eHealth and mHealth	O	O	O	O	O
standalone	O	O	O	O	O

10. Are you dealing with artificial intelligence in your workplace? *

O Yes

O No

11. Can you tell more abot this *

12. Assess your degree of optimism about the introduction of AI *

☆ ☆ ☆ ☆ ☆ ☆

13. Insert here observations or comments

12/18/2021

Figure A2. An example of the survey (second print screen).

References

1. Thrall, J.H. Teleradiology. Part I. History and clinical applications. *Radiology* **2007**, *243*, 613–617. [CrossRef] [PubMed]
2. Thrall, J.H. Teleradiology. Part II. Limitations, risks, and opportunities. *Radiology* **2007**, *244*, 325–328. [CrossRef] [PubMed]
3. Reponen, J. *Teleradiology—Changing Radiological Service Processes from Local to Regional, International and Mobile Environment*; University of Oulu: Oulu, Finland, 2010.
4. Wootton, R. Telemedicine: A cautious welcome. *BMJ* **1996**, *313*, 1375–1377. [CrossRef]
5. Giansanti, D. Teleradiology Today: The Quality Concept and the Italian Point of View. *Telemed. E-Health* **2017**, *23*, 453–455. [CrossRef] [PubMed]
6. Orlacchio, A.; Romeo, P.; Inserra, M.C.; Grigioni, M.; Giansanti, D. *Guidelines for Quality Assurance and Technical Requirements in Teleradiology*; English Translation and Revision of Rapporti ISTISAN 10/44, Rapporti ISTISAN 13/38; Istituto Superiore di Sanità: Roma, Italy, 2013; pp. 1–33.
7. Ruotsalainen, P. Privacy and security in teleradiology. *Eur. J. Radiol.* **2010**, *73*, 31–35. [CrossRef] [PubMed]
8. Giansanti, D. *Diagnostic Imaging and E-Health: Standardization, Experiences and New Opportunities*; Rapporti ISTISAN 17/10; Istituto Superiore di Sanità: Roma, Italy, 2017; pp. 1–60.
9. Giansanti, D. *Diagnostics Imaging and M-Health: Investigations on the Prospects of Integration in Cytological and Organ Diagnostics*; Rapporti ISTISAN 20/1; Istituto Superiore di Sanità: Roma, Italy, 2019; pp. 1–66.
10. Canadian Association of Radiologists. *CAR Standards for Teleradiology*; Canadian Association of Radiologists: Ottawa, ON, Canada, 2008.
11. American College of Radiology. *ACR Standard for Teleradiology*; ACR: Reston, VA, USA, 2002.
12. Teleradiology. Merrian-Webster Medical Dictionary Online. Available online: www.merriamwebster.com/medical/teleradiology (accessed on 30 September 2013).
13. Dicom, Digital Imaging and Communication in Medicine. Available online: https://www.dicomstandard.org/ (accessed on 9 January 2022).

14. Giansanti, D. The Artificial Intelligence in Digital Pathology and Digital Radiology: Where Are We? *Healthcare* **2020**, *9*, 30. [CrossRef]
15. Alsharif, M.H.; Alsharif, Y.H.; Yahya, K.; Alomari, O.A.; Albreem, M.A.; Jahid, A. Deep learning applications to combat the dissemination of COVID-19 disease: A review. *Eur. Rev. Med. Pharmacol. Sci.* **2020**, *24*, 11455–11460.
16. Ozsahin, I.; Sekeroglu, B.; Musa, M.S.; Mustapha, M.T.; Uzun Ozsahin, D. Review on Diagnosis of COVID-19 from Chest CT Images Using Artificial Intelligence. *Comput. Math. Methods Med.* **2020**, *2020*, 9756518. [CrossRef]
17. Pham, T.D. Classification of COVID-19 chest X-rays with deep learning: New models or fine tuning? *Health Inf. Sci. Syst.* **2020**, *9*, 2. [CrossRef]
18. Liang, H.; Guo, Y.; Chen, X.; Ang, K.L.; He, Y.; Jiang, N.; Du, Q.; Zeng, Q.; Lu, L.; Gao, Z.; et al. Artificial intelligence for stepwise diagnosis and monitoring of COVID-19. *Eur. Radiol.* **2022**, 1–11, Epub ahead of print. [CrossRef]
19. Stevenson, A. *Oxford Dictionary of English*, 3rd ed.; Oxford University Press: Oxford, UK, 2010.
20. Hsiang, C.W.; Lin, C.; Liu, W.C.; Lin, C.S.; Chang, W.C.; Hsu, H.H.; Huang, G.S.; Lou, Y.S.; Lee, C.C.; Wang, C.H.; et al. Detection of left ventricular systolic dysfunction using an artificial intelligence-enabled chest X-ray. *Can. J. Cardiol.* **2022**, Epub ahead of print. [CrossRef]
21. Tajik, A.J. Machine Learning for Echocardiographic imaging: Embarking on another incredible journey. *J. Am. Coll. Cardiol.* **2016**, *68*, 2296–2298. [CrossRef]
22. Krittanawong, C.; Zhang, H.; Wang, Z.; Aydar, M.; Kitai, T. Artificial intelligence in precision cardiovascular medicine. *J. Am. Coll. Cardiol.* **2017**, *69*, 2657–2664. [CrossRef] [PubMed]
23. Zhang, J.; Gajjala, S.; Agrawal, P.; Tison, G.H.; Hallock, L.A.; Beussink-Nelson, L.; Deo, R.C. Fully automated echocardiogram interpretation in clinical practice. *Circulation* **2018**, *138*, 1623–1635. [CrossRef] [PubMed]
24. Rodriguez-Ruiz, A.; Lång, K.; Gubern-Merida, A.; Broeders, M.; Gennaro, G.; Clauser, P.; Helbich, T.H.; Chevalier, M.; Tan, T.; Mertelmeier, T.; et al. Stand-Alone Artificial Intelligence for Breast Cancer Detection in Mammography: Comparison With 101 Radiologists. *J. Natl. Cancer Inst.* **2019**, *111*, 916–922. [CrossRef] [PubMed]
25. Bertini, F.; Allevi, D.; Lutero, G.; Montesi, D.; Calzà, L. Automatic Speech Classifier for Mild Cognitive Impairment and Early Dementia. *ACM Trans. Comput. Healthc.* **2022**, *3*, 1–11. [CrossRef]
26. Mak, K.K.; Pichika, M.R. Artificial intelligence in drug development: Present status and future prospects. *Drug Discov. Today* **2019**, *24*, 773–780. [CrossRef]
27. Jalal, S.; Nicolaou, S.; Parker, W. Artificial Intelligence, Radiology, and the Way Forward. *Can. Assoc. Radiol. J.* **2019**, *70*, 10–12. [CrossRef]
28. European Society of Radiology (ESR). What the radiologist should know about artificial intelligence—An ESR white paper. *Insights Imaging* **2019**, *10*, 44. [CrossRef]
29. Regulation (EU) 2017/745 of the European Parliament and of the Council of 5 April 2017 on Medical Devices, Amending Directive 2001/83/EC, Regulation (EC) No 178/2002 and Regulation (EC) No 1223/2009 and Repealing Council Directives 90/385/EEC and 93/42/EEC.2017. Available online: https://eur-lex.europa.eu/legal-content/EN/TXT/HTML/?uri=CELEX: 32017R0745&from=IT (accessed on 25 November 2021).
30. Giansanti, D. Cybersecurity and the Digital-Health: The Challenge of This Millennium. *Healthcare* **2021**, *9*, 62. [CrossRef]
31. Evidence-Based Medicine Guidelines. Available online: https://www.ebm-guidelines.com/dtk/ebmg/home (accessed on 9 January 2022).
32. Luce, B.R.; Drummond, M.; Jönsson, B.; Neumann, P.J.; Schwartz, J.S.; Siebert, U.; Sullivan, S.D. EBM, HTA, and CER: Clearing the confusion. *Milbank Q.* **2010**, *88*, 256–276. [CrossRef]
33. McGlynn, E.A.; Kosecoff, J.; Brook, R.H. Format and conduct of consensus development conferences. Multi-nation comparison. *Int. J. Technol. Assess. Health Care* **1990**, *6*, 450–469. [CrossRef]
34. Eddy, D.M. Evidence-Based Medicine: A Unified Approach. *Health Affairs* **2005**, *24*, 9–17. [CrossRef] [PubMed]
35. National Library of Medicine. Available online: https://pubmed.ncbi.nlm.nih.gov/?term=%28acceptance%29+AND+%2 8artificial+intelligence%5BTitle%2FAbstract%5D%29+AND+Radiology&sort=date&size=200 (accessed on 9 January 2022).
36. National Library of Medicine. Available online: https://pubmed.ncbi.nlm.nih.gov/?term=%28%28consensus%29+AND+ %28artificial+intelligence%5BTitle%2FAbstract%5D%29%29+AND+%28radiology%5BTitle%2FAbstract%5D%29&sort=date& size=200 (accessed on 9 January 2022).
37. Lennartz, S.; Dratsch, T.; Zopfs, D.; Persigehl, T.; Maintz, D.; Hokamp, N.G.; Dos Santos, D.P. Use and Control of Artificial Intelligence in Patients Across the Medical Workflow: Single-Center Questionnaire Study of Patient Perspectives. *J. Med. Internet Res.* **2021**, *23*, e24221. [CrossRef] [PubMed]
38. Zhang, Z.; Citardi, D.; Wang, D.; Genc, Y.; Shan, J.; Fan, X. Patients' perceptions of using artificial intelligence (AI)-based technology to comprehend radiology imaging data. *Health Inform. J.* **2021**, *27*, 14604582211011215. [CrossRef]
39. Ongena, Y.P.; Haan, M.; Yakar, D.; Kwee, T.C. Patients' views on the implementation of artificial intelligence in radiology: Development and validation of a standardized questionnaire. *Eur. Radiol.* **2020**, *30*, 1033–1040. [CrossRef] [PubMed]
40. Hendrix, N.; Hauber, B.; Lee, C.I.; Bansal, A.; Veenstra, D.L. Artificial intelligence in breast cancer screening: Primary care provider preferences. *J. Am. Med. Inform. Assoc.* **2021**, *28*, 1117–1124. [CrossRef]
41. Abuzaid, M.M.; Elshami, W.; McConnell, J.; Tekin, H.O. An extensive survey on radiographers from the Middle East and India on artificial intelligence integration in radiology practice. *Health Technol.* **2021**, *11*, 1045–1050. [CrossRef]

42. Abuzaid, M.M.; Tekin, H.O.; Reza, M.; Elhag, I.R.; Elshami, W. Assessment of MRI technologists in acceptance and willingness to integrate artificial intelligence into practice. *Radiography* **2021**, *27*, S83–S87. [CrossRef]
43. Giansanti, D.; Rossi, I.; Monoscalco, L. Lessons from the COVID-19 Pandemic on the Use of Artificial Intelligence in Digital Radiology: The Submission of a Survey to Investigate the Opinion of Insiders. *Healthcare* **2021**, *9*, 331. [CrossRef] [PubMed]
44. Abuzaid, M.M.; Elshami, W.; Tekin, H.; Issa, B. Assessment of the Willingness of Radiologists and Radiographers to Accept the Integration of Artificial Intelligence into Radiology Practice. *Acad. Radiol.* **2020**, *29*, 87–94. [CrossRef] [PubMed]
45. Alelyani, M.; Alamri, S.; Alqahtani, M.S.; Musa, A.; Almater, H.; Alqahtani, N.; Alshahrani, F.; Alelyani, S. Radiology Community Attitude in Saudi Arabia about the Applications of Artificial Intelligence in Radiology. *Healthcare* **2021**, *9*, 834. [CrossRef] [PubMed]
46. European Society of Radiology (ESR). Impact of artificial intelligence on radiology: A EuroAIM survey among members of the European Society of Radiology. *Insights Imaging* **2019**, *10*, 105. [CrossRef] [PubMed]
47. Galán, G.C.; Portero, F.S. Medical students' perceptions of the impact of artificial intelligence in Radiology. *Radiologia* **2021**, in press. [CrossRef]
48. Aldosari, B. User acceptance of a picture archiving and communication system (PACS) in a Saudi Arabian hospital radiology department. *BMC Med. Inform. Decis. Mak.* **2012**, *12*, 44. [CrossRef]
49. Moss, R.J.; Süle, A.; Kohl, S. eHealth and mHealth. *Eur. J. Hosp. Pharm.* **2019**, *26*, 57–58. [CrossRef] [PubMed]
50. Shan, H.; Padole, A.; Homayounieh, F.; Kruger, U.; Khera, R.D.; Nitiwarangkul, C.; Kalra, M.K.; Wang, G. Competitive performance of a modularized deep neural network compared to commercial algorithms for low-dose CT image reconstruction. *Nat. Mach. Intell.* **2019**, *1*, 269–276. [CrossRef]
51. Moher, D.; Altman, D.G.; Schulz, K.F.; Simera, I.; Wager, E. (Eds.) Guidelines for Reporting Health Research: A User's Manual. Available online: https://onlinelibrary.wiley.com/doi/abs/10.1002/9781118715598.ch20 (accessed on 9 January 2022).
52. Ministero Della Salute Rivede Elenco Società Scientifiche per Stesura Linee Guida. 41 Società in Più. Available online: http://www.aiponet.it/news/104-ufficio-stampa/2149-ministero-della-salute-rivede-elenco-societa-scientifiche-per-stesura-linee-guida-41-societa-in-piu.html (accessed on 9 January 2022).
53. Federazione Delle Società Medico-Scientifiche Italiane. Available online: https://portale.fism.it/ (accessed on 9 January 2022).
54. Federazione Delle Associazioni Scientifiche dei Tecnici di Radiologia. Available online: https://www.associazionefaster.org/ (accessed on 9 January 2022).
55. Federazione Delle Associazioni Scientifiche e Tecniche. Available online: https://fast.mi.it/chi-siamo/ (accessed on 9 January 2022).
56. Thomassin-Naggara, I.; Balleyguier, C.; Ceugnart, L.; Heid, P.; Lenczner, G.; Maire, A.; Séradour, B.; Verzaux, L.; Taourel, P. Conseil National Professionnel de la Radiologie et Imagerie Médicale (G4). Artificial intelligence and breast screening: French Radiology Community position paper. *Diagn. Interv. Imaging* **2019**, *100*, 553–566. [CrossRef]
57. Avanzo, M.; Trianni, A.; Botta, F.; Talamonti, C.; Stasi, M.; Iori, M. Artificial Intelligence and the Medical Physicist: Welcome to the Machine. *Appl. Sci.* **2021**, *11*, 1691. [CrossRef]
58. Coppola, F.; Faggioni, L.; Regge, D.; Giovagnoni, A.; Golfieri, R.; Bibbolino, C.; Miele, V.; Neri, E.; Grassi, R. Artificial intelligence: Radiologists' expectations and opinions gleaned from a nationwide online survey. *Radiol. Med.* **2021**, *126*, 63–71. [CrossRef]
59. Diaz, O.; Guidi, G.; Ivashchenko, O.; Colgan, N.; Zanca, F. Artificial intelligence in the medical physics community: An international survey. *Phys. Med.* **2021**, *81*, 141–146. [CrossRef]

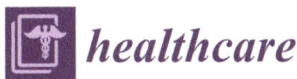

Commentary

Artificial Intelligence in Digital Pathology: What Is the Future? Part 1: From the Digital Slide Onwards

Maria Rosaria Giovagnoli [1] and Daniele Giansanti [2,*]

[1] Faculty of Medicine and Psychology, Sapienza University, Piazzale Aldo Moro, 00185 Roma, Italy; mr.giovagnoli.univ.sap@hotmail.com
[2] Centre Tisp, Istituto Superiore di Sanità, 00161 Roma, Italy
* Correspondence: daniele.giansanti@iss.it; Tel.: +39-06-49902701

Abstract: This commentary aims to address the field of *Artificial intelligence* (AI) in *Digital Pathology* (DP) both in terms of the global situation and research perspectives. It has four polarities. *First*, it revisits the evolutions of digital pathology with particular care to the two fields of the digital cytology and the digital histology. *Second*, it illustrates the main fields in the employment of AI in DP. *Third*, it looks at the future directions of the research challenges from both a clinical and technological point of view. *Fourth*, it discusses the transversal problems among these challenges and implications and introduces the immediate work to implement.

Keywords: e-health; medical devices; m-health; digital-pathology; picture archive and communication system; artificial intelligence; cytology; histology

1. Introduction

Diagnostic pathology has undergone important changes and leaps forward by means of digitalization, which have allowed, from time to time, on the one hand, important changes in decision-making processes, and on the other, important changes in *workflow* and therefore in the *job description* of the insiders [1,2].

All this has had an important impact on the organization of work from one side and on the training of the figures involved in the activities on the other, having to prepare them to make the necessary changes to adapt them to the ever-changing *job description* and interactions with the tools (optics/mechatronics/informatics) in ever-more rapid obsolescence and gradually being more and more able to integrate with *eHealth* and *mHealth* [1–6].

We are moving from physical storage systems of slides to virtual storage of virtual-slides (i.e., *e-slides* or *digital-slides*) [3].

Old problems such as the organization of physical storage spaces are giving way to new problems such as physical (conservative) data security and cybersecurity.

Now there is less talk of archives and multi-archives for slides and more and more of how many petabytes or exabytes will be needed for the *e-slides*.

The changes have been so rapid that someone is starting to ask the fateful question: Will the microscope still be needed as we know it today?

We can undoubtedly highlight how, to date, diagnostic pathology has gone through two important revolutions.

The great *innovations* in the field of the diagnostic pathology involved first the introduction of the immune-histo-chemistry in 1980 and second in the introduction of *next-generation sequencing for cancer diagnostics* around 2010.

The *first revolution* involved the introduction of digital pathology and therefore of the key elements from the *e-slide*, up to the acquisition system (video-camera or scanner) and to archiving system, the picture archive and communication system (PACS) for digital pathology [3].

This *second revolution*, if we leave out the era of robotic telepathology (which does not seem to have had a great impact in pathological diagnostics), had two important moments that we can call (a) the *revolution of digital pathology in eHealth* [5] with the possibility of accessing from the personal computer to PACS servers through virtual microscopy and (b) the *revolution of digital pathology in mHealth* [1] with the possibility of accessing the same servers from smartphones and tablets through a virtual microscope. As it has been highlighted by M Avanzo et al. in the review [6], nowadays, AI shows (1) the potentiality to access and correlate large amount of data and (2) direct prospective in the world of diagnostics.

Regarding (1), it is highlighted that today [6], both radiological and pathology images are stored in the PACS; moreover, with the introduction of electronic health records (EHRs), systematic collections of patient health information have been made available, which include both qualitative data, medical records, and laboratory and diagnostics information. AI, if applied to these big digital stores, could prove useful for epidemiological, clinical, and research studies.

Scientists in DP could benefit of AI from combining histopathological data obtained, analyzed, and shared with other sources of clinical data such as that obtained from omics and/or other databases with clinical data/demographic data and/or sources with BIG-DATA.

With regard to (2), it is highlighted that the development of the digital pathology [6] due to the introduction of whole-slide scanners and the progression of computer vision algorithms have significantly grown the usage of AI to perform tumor diagnosis, subtyping, grading, staging, and prognostic prediction. In the big-data era, the pathological diagnosis of the future could merge proteomics and genomics.

It is evident that AI is clearly helping to integrate information from multiple sources.

Furthermore, neural networks from AI are used, for example, to extract pertinent details from written notes from the slide representation.

In general, all of us are also expecting AI in DP as a deus ex machina to diminish the error rate and optimize the time of work.

2. Purpose

The contribution is in line with the Special Issue "The Artificial Intelligence in Digital Pathology and Digital Radiology: Where Are We?" https://www.mdpi.com/journal/healthcare/special_issues/AI_Digital_Pathology_Radiology (6 July 2021) [6].

The aim is to highlight, in light of the foregoing, the important aspects of the transitions towards DP and AI, highlighting: (a) the lights and shadows relating to the introduction of AI based on DP and (b) what could be the future directions to face to stabilize the AI in DP.

3. The Revolution of the Digital Slide

The introduction of *digital slides* (*e-slide* or *virtual-slide*) is undoubtedly a revolutionary change for the pathologist, comparable to that of the introduction of *google maps* for *cartography*.

Through digital pathology, it is in fact possible to navigate through the *e-slide* with reference to coordinates, perform *Zoom and Pan* operations and set references just as with *Google Maps*. Historically, DP in the first applications was faced with implementing telepathology connections [3]. In the first phases, there was talk of *telepathology* and not of DP. Conceptually, there were and still there are two methods to face *telepathology* (TP): *static TP* and *dynamic TP*. Static TP consists of the capture and digitalization of images selected by a pathologist or pathologist assistant, which are then transmitted remotely through electronic means. *Dynamic TP* consists of the direct communication between two different centers by using microscopes equipped with a *tele-robotic system* oriented to explore the slide, remotely operated by the *tele-pathologist* or an *assistant tele-pathologist* to reach a remote diagnosis. As an alternative solution between the two methods, widely increased, year after year, there is the *virtual microscopy* (*VM*) starting from the first applications. The latter does not refer to the *tele-control of microscopes*, whilst the glass is scanned as a whole, producing an *e-slide*, and a pathologist or the assistant pathologist can navigate remotely (via internet) inside this *e-slide* or *virtual slide* in a manner akin to a real microscope. It has to be considered that a single file representing the *e-slide* for pathology applications could reach several tens of gigabytes, more than in the case of applications of digital echography. Thus, the design of an appropriate visualization strategy is a basic core aspect.

Today, the diffusion of the VM was helped by: (a) the availability of fast internet connections; (b) the availability of consolidated visualization strategies; (c) the availability of power image acquisition cameras/scanners; (d) the availability of free visualization software.

We can clearly consider today that VM is an integral part of DP. Therefore, it can be used in biomedical laboratories with great potential. This can affect the organization of work and has the potential to change and improve training [2,4].

DP is not only *digital slides* [6]. However, it is impossible not to point out that *digital slides/e-slides* are a large part of DP.

For this reason, it is important to highlight some strategic aspects of this discipline of the VM and to consider how they evolved over the time.

3.1. The Difference between the Digital Cytology and Digital Histology

The cytologist and the histologist interact differently with the slides; therefore, when moving to the digital world, this aspect must be strongly considered. The cytologist analyses the cell while the histologist analyses the tissue. If we can make a comparison with architecture, the cytologist focuses on the brick and looks inside, whilst the histologist looks at the entire wall. For the cytologist to look inside the cell, it is particularly important to use the focus function, which is not needed by the histologist. This translates into cytology in an important need for digitization: that of allowing the focus function in the digital world. This is implemented with the creation of different digital layers to simulate fire through the *Z-stack* [3] function or other solutions that currently do not allow automatic implementation [7]. For these reasons, the *e-slide* in cytology requires an exorbitant memory occupation to cope with the *Z-stack*.

3.2. The Two Steps of the Revolution of the Digital Pathology: Integration into eHealth and mHealth

When we refer to the introduction of digital pathology, we must duly consider that there have been two important phases synchronized with the evolution of ICT that in healthcare have led to the developments of *eHealth* and *mHealth* applications.

Consequently, the first *client-server* informatic buildings had, in the era of *eHealth* developments, a strong component based on architectures based on PCs that connected via LAN/WAN.

Figure 1 shows an example of PC access to a *virtual slide* in the case of digital cytology.

Subsequently, starting with the release in 2008 of the first smartphones and/or tablets as we know them today [1], digital pathology has begun to find a fertile vehicle in *mHealth*.

Figure 2 highlights a first application in *mHealth* in digital cytology with the Nokia c6 with the operative system Symbian (Symbian Ltd., Southwark UK) device, a border element between mobile phones and smartphones in a WI-FI hotspot.

Figure 3, again with reference to digital cytology, reports some accesses in *mHealth* by a tablet (A), from a train without WI-FI, and in other situations via smartphone (B).

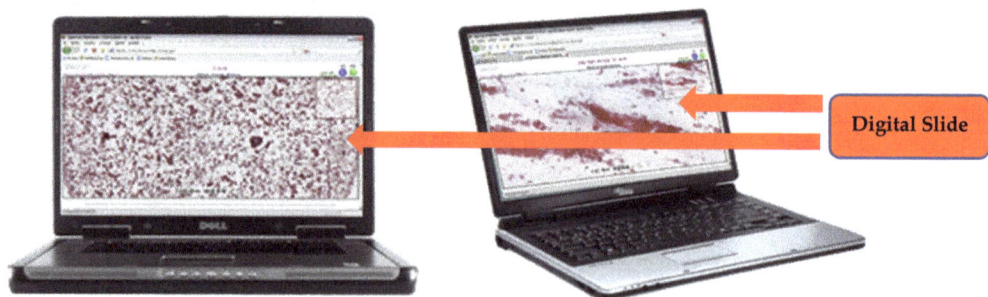

Figure 1. Access to the digital slides using eHealth.

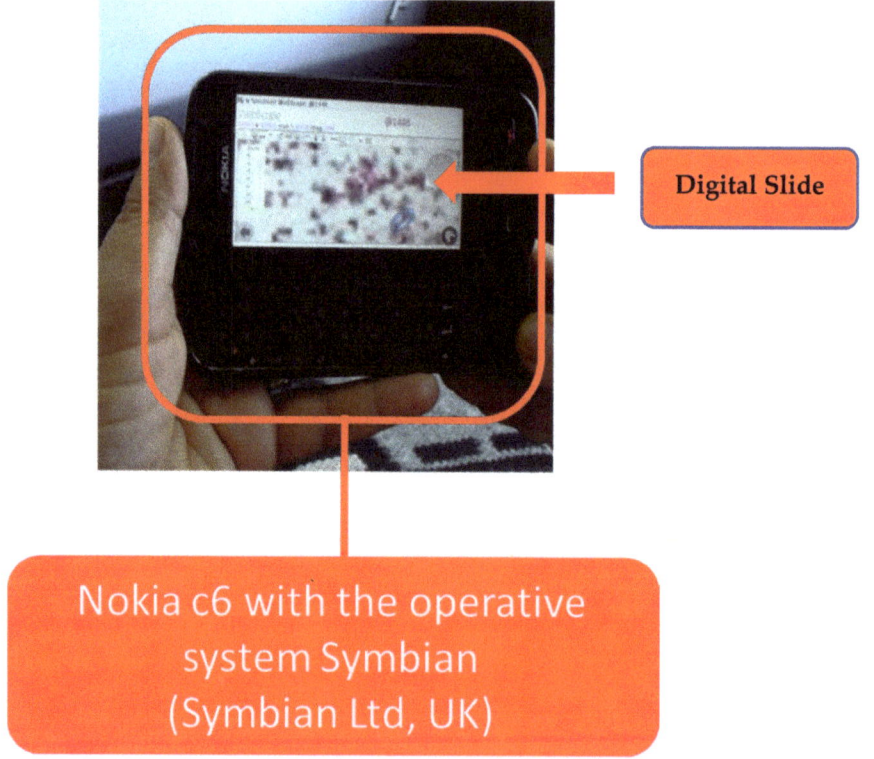

Figure 2. Access to the digital slides using mHealth not using the smartphone.

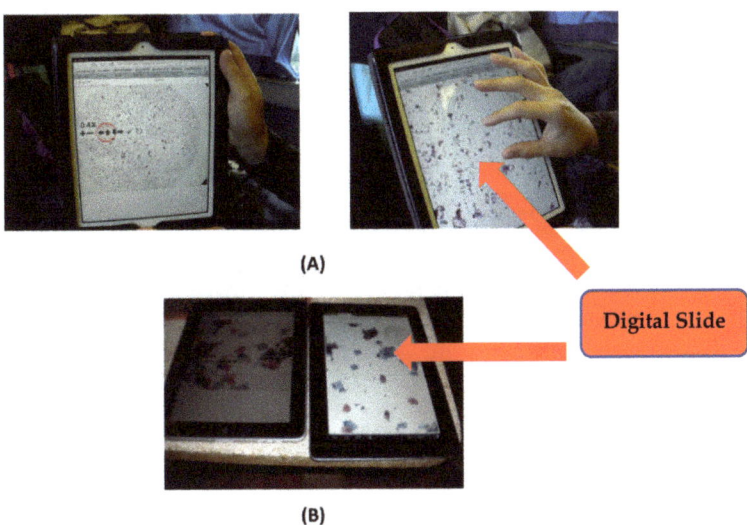

Figure 3. Access to the digital slides using mHealth (**A**) while navigating by a train without Wi-Fi; (**B**) a static connection.

3.3. The Acceptance of the Introduction: The HTA Studies Based on Properly Designed Surveys

A strategic aspect in the introduction of a technology is that of acceptance. Important aspects can be overlooked; moreover, problems of interaction with technologies that depend on generations could also arise. For example, the cytologist while navigating with the traditional microscope has a way of navigating and noticing important details with the side of the eyeball facing outward like that of primitive man to protect himself from attacks by ferocious predators. Switching to a PC-based method in *eHealth* first and *mHealth* on a smartphone or tablet later determines a radical change. Therefore, it is necessary to carry out targeted studies on the acceptance of technologies, focused on the actors, with reference to the most critical applications, as in the case of digital cytology. In the study reported in [5], we highlighted the importance of a health technology assessment approach based on a survey centred on the figures involved from a working point of view in digital cytology (which, as we have seen, presents major problems) in the *eHealth* phase. In the study reported in [1], we highlighted the importance of a health technology assessment approach with a similar configuration in the *mHealth* phase.

3.4. The Potentialities in the e-Learning/Remote Training

There is no one who does not see, in the COVID-19 era, that DP has important advantages in training regarding social distancing and the lightening of laboratories. Today, it is possible to access large databases and select targeted e-slide-based studies. Just to give an example, Leeds also has important archives with free access to the site https://www.virtualpathology.leeds.ac.uk/, accessed on 6 July 2021, [8].

See one of the many studies directly navigable with your browser in *eHealth* or *mHealth* by accessing the dedicated archive https://www.virtualpathology.leeds.ac.uk/slides/library/, accessed on 6 July 2021, [9], having fun with one of the many digital slides when navigating using a virtual microscope and simple mouse clicks https://www.virtualpathology.leeds.ac.uk/slides/library/view.php?path=%2FResearch_4%2FTeaching%2FEducation%2FManchester_FRCPath%2FDN%2F124388.svs, accessed on 6 July 2021, [10].

In teaching, we highlighted the possibility of setting two important approaches [2]: (a) that of using very large tablets such as LIMS whiteboards or other ones in a finger-based and cooperative way to navigate virtual slides (Figure 4A), and (b) the other one based on a slide viewer or scope system with a webcam and a network transmitter to tablet/smartphone, even when not present (Figure 4B), such as, for example, the DMshare system (Leica Microsystems Co., Nussloch GmbH, Germany). Both have allowed to free up important resources in this pandemic period, such as dedicated laboratories. Of course, today, we can add a third dedicated method: one based on video conferencing with screen sharing.

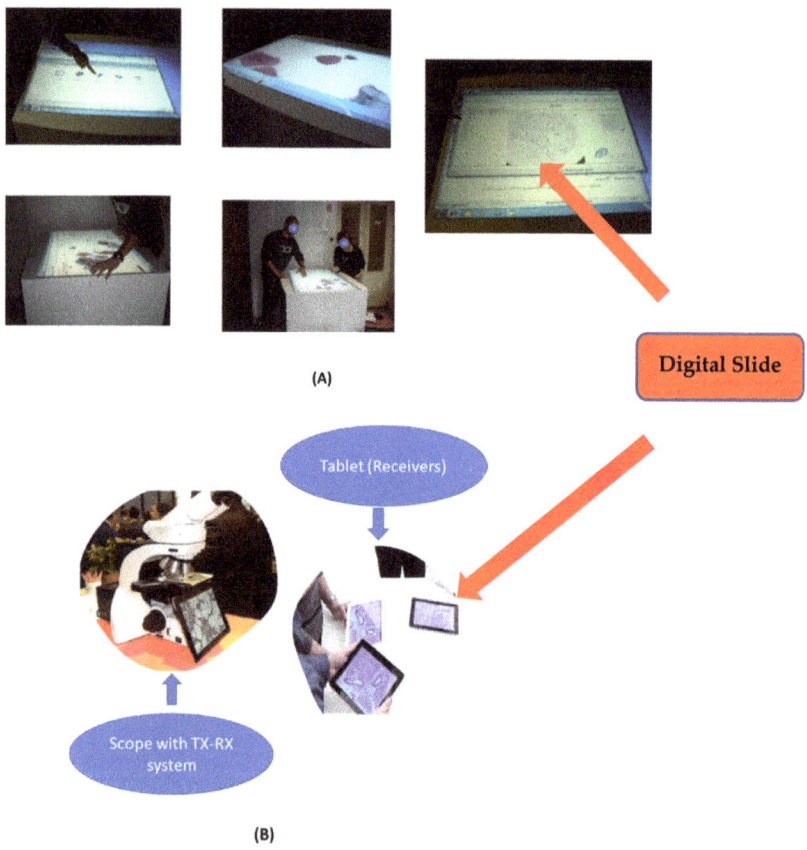

Figure 4. The two different types of training: (**A**) using a very large tablet; (**B**) using the DMSHARE.

3.5. The Standardization: A Slower Standardization Rate When Compared to Digital Radiology

The standardization of imaging in PD has had and is having a more tortuous road than digital radiology, wherein, thanks to DICOM, since the 1990s [11], a rapid process of digitization and compatibility of the diagnostic tools of the organs and functions has been initiated (echo, NMR, CT, PET, etc.).

Standardization in this area started with a slower process, and consequently, the compatibility between different manufacturers towards the standard has been delayed [6].

Today, DICOM WSI http://dicom.nema.org/Dicom/DICOMWSI/, accessed on 6 July 2021, [12] is used as standard in DP.

This standard considers the *whole slide images* (WSI)s in DP.

These images are exceptionally large.

As described in [12], a typical sample may be 20 mm × 15 mm in size and may be digitized with a resolution of 0.25 micrometers/pixel (conventionally described as *microns per pixel*, or *mpp*); here in the following we recall the characteristics reported in [12].

Most optical microscopes have an eyepiece which provides 10×magnification, so using a 40× objective lens results in 400× magnification.

Although instruments that digitize microscope slides do not use an eyepiece and may not use microscope objective lenses, by convention, images captured with a resolution of 0.25 mpp are referred to as 40×, images captured with a resolution of 0.5 mpp are referred to as 20X, etc.

The resulting image is therefore about 80,000 × 60,000 pixels, or 4.8 Gp.

Images are usually captured with 24-bit color, so the image data size is about 15GB.

This is a typical example, but larger images may be captured. Sample sizes up to 50 mm × 25 mm may be captured from conventional 1 × 3 slides, and even larger samples may exist on 2 × 3 slides.

Images may be digitized at resolutions higher than 0.25 mpp; some scanning instruments now support oil immersion lenses, which can magnify up to 100×, yielding 0.1 mpp resolution. Some operations described in [12] may further enlarge the data occupancy [12].

For example, a sample of 50 mm × 25 mm could be captured at 0.1 mpp with 10 Z-planes in the Z-stack, yielding a stack of 10 images of dimension 500,000 × 250,000 pixels. *Each plane would contain 125 Gp, or 375 GB of data, and the entire image dataset would contain a staggering 3.75 TB of data.*

4. Towards the Revolution of the Digital Pathology and Artificial Intelligence

4.1. What Is Emerging in the Application of the Artificial Intelligence in Digital Pathology

We carried out research with the aim of identifying the work to be completed, in terms of challenges and opportunities, towards stabilizing the use of artificial intelligence in DP, and then integrating what is highlighted with the considerations on digital pathology that we carried out in the previous section.

A quick look at PubMed with the following search key:

(*digital pathology* [Title]) AND (*artificial intelligence* [Title]) currently reports 17 works [6,13–28].

Among these works, one respects the search rule:

(digital pathology [Title]) AND (artificial intelligence [Title]) AND (COVID-19) [20] that is, it relates to COVID-19.

What is highlighted by these works (many of which are editorial and/or opinion) from a general point of view are the following aspects. The first aspect is that when scholars talk about artificial intelligence in digital pathology, they refer more to the aspects of imaging and essentially histological imaging. The second aspect is that scholars begin to identify interesting perspectives—for example, in oncology [15,25] or in toxicology [14,24]. The last aspect, in line with our objective, is that scholars are interrogating the work to be completed in a prospective way [25–28].

Important perspectives have been identified for example:

- Through a review [15] on immuno-oncology.
- In a Special Issue [14] and in an opinion article [24] of a working group in pathological diagnostics in toxicology.
- Through a report [22] for the prediction of positive lymph nodes from primary tumors in bladder cancer.
- In cancer staging [18], it is well known that recent AI approaches have been applied to pathology images toward diagnostic, prognostic, and treatment prediction-related tasks in cancer. AI approaches according to this study [18] have the potential to overcome the limitations of conventional TNM staging and tumor grading approaches, providing a direct prognostic prediction of disease outcome independent of tumor stage and grade.

In the review that we have preselected as the only study linked to COVID-19 [20], it is highlighted that the effects of COVID-19 on research and clinical trials have also been significant with changes to protocols, suspensions of studies and the redeployment of resources to COVID-19 also useful for the applications of AI in DP. In this article, the authors explore the specific impact of COVID-19 on clinical and academic pathology and explore how digital pathology and artificial intelligence can play a key role in safeguarding clinical services and pathology-based research in the current climate and in the future.

We have identified *four prospective studies* that identify the critical issues and the work to be carried out [25–28].

The first study, although [25] it is not a review but an opinion, clearly identifies and discusses the critical issues in precision oncology by identifying some points on which to focus attention. The study aimed to provide a broad framework for incorporating AI and machine learning tools into clinical oncology, with an emphasis on biomarker development. *They discussed some of the challenges related to the use of AI, including the need for well-curated validation datasets, regulatory approval, and fair reimbursement strategies.*

The second study is an interesting review on the critical issues and the work still to be completed to arrive at the clinical routine [26]. This work highlights that while this is an exciting development that could discover novel predictive clinical information and potentially address international pathology workforce shortages, there is a clear need for a robust and evidence-based framework in which to develop these new tools in a collaborative manner that meets regulatory approval. *With these issues in mind, they have set out a roadmap to help academia, industry, and clinicians develop new software tools to the point of approved clinical use.*

The third study is an interesting review [27] that highlights that the advent of whole-slide imaging (WSI), the availability of faster networks, and cheaper storage solutions have made it easier for pathologists to manage digital slide images and share them for clinical use. In parallel, unprecedented advances in machine learning have enabled the synergy of artificial intelligence and digital pathology, which offers image-based diagnosis possibilities that were once limited only to radiology and cardiology. Integration of digital slides into the pathology workflow, advanced algorithms, and computer-aided diagnostic techniques extend the frontiers of the pathologist's view beyond a microscopic slide and enable true utilization and integration of knowledge in new manner; therefore, it is important to focus on the WSI, now standardized in DICOM WSI and as radiologists and cardiologists move in line with the standards.

The fourth study is an interesting review [28] where the authors provide a realistic account of all the challenges of adopting AI algorithms in digital pathology from both engineering and pathology perspectives.

In the work, we found an interesting and shareable outline of the challenges of AI in digital pathology that naturally recalls what emerges in the other three interesting prospective studies [25–28] and lends itself well to the objectives of our study.

4.2. What Are the Perfectives and the Work to Be Carried out to Fully Integrate Artificial Intelligence in Digital Pathology?

4.2.1. The Guiding Approach

In Section 3, we highlighted the characteristics and criticalities of the digital pathology on which the AI will have to rely and, in particular, which ones will have to be taken into account in routine applications.

We have, furthermore, seen above that to make AI a consolidated reality in digital pathology, it is necessary: (a) proceed with standardization processes including the need for well-curated validation datasets, regulatory approval and fair reimbursement strategies [25], (b) define roadmaps to help academia, industry, and clinicians to develop new software tools to the point of approved clinical use through concerted actions [26], (c) focus on the WSI, now standardized in DICOM WSI and, as the radiologists and cardiologists move in line with the DICOM standards [27], (d) provide a realistic account of all challenges of adopting AI algorithms in digital pathology from both engineering and pathology perspectives [28].

4.2.2. Future Challenges

In their exhaustive review, Hamid Reza Tizhoosh and Liron Pantanowitz [28] recently categorized the challenges to be faced and also the evident opportunities. We fully share this useful approach organized as a useful grid. We summarize this briefly, referring to the review for an in-depth view.

Challenges in AI in Digital Pathology

The challenges that digital pathology presents for the integration of AI have been identified in [28]'s 10 *challenges* (Figure 5, table in the left):

1. *Lack of labeled data*

    The AI algorithms require a large set of good-quality training images. These training images must ideally be "labeled" (i.e., annotated). This is not easily feasible in DP.

2. *Pervasive variability*

    There are several basic types of tissue (e.g., epithelium, connective tissue, nervous tissue, and muscle). The actual number of patterns derived from these tissues from a computational point of view is nearly infinite if the histopathology images are to be "understood" by computer algorithms.

3. *Non-Boolean nature of diagnostic tasks*

    In pathology, not all can be summarized into two possible values such as "yes" or "no" (e.g., benign, or malignant). This is a too drastic a simplification of the complex nature of the diagnosis in this field. However, today, this is really not an issue; indeed, discrete variables (e.g., 1, 2, 3, 4) can be managed by machine learning, and there are also available methods based on regression machine learning for continuous variables, as reported in [29], for example.

4. *Dimensionality obstacle*

    As we have highlighted in Section 3, the WSI deals with gigapixel digital images of extremely large dimensions up to 3.75 TB. Deep ANNs used in AI act on much smaller image dimensions (i.e., not larger than 350 by 350 pixels).

5. *Turing test dilemma*

    The pathologist has the last word on the decision process when AI solutions are integrated in the workflow. Thus, full automation is probably neither possible, it seems, nor wise, as the Turing test postulates.

6. *Uni-task orientation of weak artificial intelligence*

    What we consider today is mostly "weak AI" in contrast with strong AI, also called artificial general intelligence (AGI). Deep ANNs belong to the class of weak AI algorithms, as they are designed to perform only one task. Therefore, we need to separately train multiple AI solutions for different tasks. This obviously has implications.

7. *Affordability of required computational expenses*

    Solutions with AI use graphical processing units (GPUs), highly specialized electronic circuits for fast processing of pixel-based data (i.e., digital images and graphics). These devices are expensive, and their adoption needs specific financial programs.

8. *Adversarial attacks—The noise in the deep decisions*

    This is a common problem in AI; a little change in a pixel, for example, due to the noise may cause a completely different output in the ANN.

9. *Lack of transparency and interoperability*

The major drawbacks of artificial neural networks (ANN)s when used as classifiers is the lack of interoperability and transparency. Some consider ANNs to enclose a "black box" after the training.

10. *Realism of artificial intelligence*

There is currently optimism about the opportunities of ANNs, as has been highlighted above in the studies [13–28]. There are several difficulties with deploying AI tools in practice depending on the expectance and the objectives of the pathologist. There is no doubt that three are the preliminary requirements to improve this: (1) ease of use, (2) financial return on investment connected to the application, and (3) trust (such as, for example, the accountable performances).

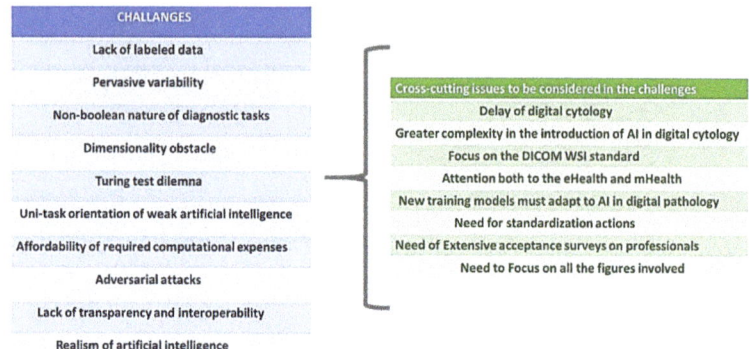

Figure 5. The challenges and cross-cutting issues emerging in the application of AI in DP.

Further Cross-Cutting Issues

We agree with the categorization identified by Hamid Reza Tizhoosh and Liron Pantanowitz [28], and I believe that it can be used as a reference for evaluating the future efforts of AI in digital pathology. Without introducing new challenges in detail, we would like to integrate the analysis with what emerged in Section 3 and in the other three selected prospective studies discussed above [25–28].

There are in fact aspects to be highlighted that act in a transversal way and are decisive for facing the 10 challenges identified in the categorization.

Cross-cutting issues to be considered in the challenges (Figure 5, table in the right).

N1. *Delay of digital cytology.* We have seen in Section 3 how digital pathology in digital imaging includes the two macro-sectors of digital histology and digital cytology. We have also seen above how in the studies addressed we refer mainly to the world of digital histology. This naturally translates into a foreseeable future delay of digital cytology due to less dedication on the part of scholars.

N2. *Greater complexity in the introduction of AI in digital cytology.* We highlighted in Section 3 that digital cytology needs the emulation of the focus function "to break through the sample"; this translates into the need to introduce the Z-stack, which can increase the WSI even 100 times compared to the histological case (up to 3.75 TB). This aspect must be duly considered.

N3. *Focus on the DICOM WSI standard.* As highlighted in [27], it is necessary to keep in mind the recent releases of standards to face large-scale studies on the introduction of AI in digital pathology and take inspiration from the world of digital radiology and cardiology, where the DICOM standards are now customary. This must apply to both digital histology and digital cytology. The weak AI mentioned above in *challenge 6* must navigate in extraction starting from standard WSI also to act on *challenge 10*, relating to concreteness and realism.

N4. *Attention both to eHealth and mHealth.* For AI, we need to consider both the worlds of *eHealth* and *mHealth*, where DP has stabilized through a path of acceptance [1,5].

N5. *New training models must adapt to AI in digital pathology.* Training models based on WSI and tablets and smartphones being remotely used must be able to include the provision of training also on *AI-based packages* and approaches. In this way, it is possible to integrate the two worlds of digital pathology and AI already in the training phase [2,4].

N6. *Need for standardization actions.* On the one hand, there is a need for manufacturers to adapt to standards [12]. On the other hand, as happens and/or is happening for telemedicine/tele-rehabilitation and alternative rehabilitation based on robotics, it is necessary to start a formal integration of digital pathology services connected with AI, as highlighted in [6]. This formal integration must have: a first step for consensus/acceptance paths between professionals that leads to important guidelines or recommendations. A second step that includes the provision of services in the healthcare offers the portfolio with coding of the service and reimbursement.

N7. *Need of extensive acceptance surveys on professionals.* This too is an important aspect interconnected with the previous ones. In Section 3, we highlighted how in the two phases of the introduction of digital pathology—*eHealth* and *mHealth*— there were important acceptance studies using HTA methods conducted on professionals through specific surveys [1,5]. These studies are also important in view of possible consensus conferences, or the activation of study groups dedicated to the activities of the previous points.

N8. *Need to focus on all the figures involved.* The introduction of AI in DP revolves various working figures in addition to the pathologist. These are the workers who will be involved in the reorganization of workflows, such as the clinical engineer and the biomedical laboratory technician [4,5]. These figures must be involved in standardization studies.

5. Conclusions and Work in Progress

5.1. The Evidences in the Study

In this study, the introduction of artificial intelligence in digital pathology was addressed. The study first tackled the second revolution in diagnostic pathology determined by the introduction of digital pathology techniques [1–6]. There is no doubt that most of the applications of AI take place in diagnostic imaging and that, therefore, AI rests on the imaging techniques used in digital pathology.

In analysing the important aspects of digital pathology, some important points/steps were noted:

- *The difference between digital cytology and digital histology.*
- *The two steps of the revolution of the digital pathology: integration into eHealth and mHealth.*
- *The acceptance of the introduction: the HTA studies based on designed surveys.*
- *The potentialities in the e-learning/remote training.*
- *The standardization: a slower standardization rate when compared to digital radiology.*

We then questioned the state of the next revolution that is anticipated due to the introduction of AI in DP. Through an overview of some important studies, some important development guidelines have been identified and, in line with the objectives of this study, the challenges to be addressed in detail and the transversal problems as they emerge both from the overview and from the characteristics and problems of digital pathology highlighted in the section dedicated to this discipline. The *10 challenges* were therefore recalled, starting from the grid identified in [28], and eight emerged transversal issues to be considered in these challenges were introduced and discussed (Figure 5).

5.2. Actual Developments and Future Work

All that is highlighted in the *cross-cutting issues* is, in a certain sense, of strong scientific interest and needs attention if we think of a routine introduction of AI in digital pathology. A point where we intend to contribute is that (no. 7) relating to acceptance based on surveys on key figures (no. 8), which is preparatory to standardization actions (no. 6 and no. 3–4). Inheriting the experience gained from previous studies [1,5], in which we had developed paper surveys for this purpose (relating to the introduction of digital pathology first in eHealth and then in mHealth), we are developing an electronic survey as a tool to be used with this purpose and we are using it to investigate this.

5.3. Limitations of the Study

The overview in the section was conducted with the search key "Artificial Intelligence", wanting to stay on a higher and general level regarding the topic in line with the objectives of the study. Other more specific searches can be executed on aspects of a lower hierarchical level such as those relating to the algorithms of use. Artificial intelligence uses a myriad of different methodologies, techniques, and approaches that deserve specific review and research extended to non-medical databases, even if we are dealing with medical problems.

A long discussion deserves a targeted approach in the collection of *medical knowledge* in this area relating to supervised ANNs and unsupervised ANNs to collect successful and/or unsuccessful experiences.

A key search, for example, limited to the medical database PubMed of (digital pathology [Title]) AND (deep learning [Title]) led, at the date of this study, to 14 results [30], of which one was included in the one we made.

Another example of research on the same database of (digital pathology [Title]) AND (machine learning [Title]) led, at the date of this study, to seven results [31], of which four were included in the one we made above.

Such a research is more closely related to the specific performance of algorithms in DP and can highlight important development opportunities that must certainly be taken into account in any wide-ranging reviews.

Author Contributions: Conceptualization, D.G. and M.R.G.; methodology, D.G.; software, D.G.; validation, D.G. and M.R.G.; formal analysis, All; investigation, All; resources, All; data curation, D.G.; writing—original draft preparation, D.G.; writing—review and editing, All; visualization, All; supervision, All; project administration, All; funding acquisition, none. All authors have read and agreed to the published version of the manuscript.

Funding: This research received no external funding.

Institutional Review Board Statement: Not applicable.

Informed Consent Statement: Not applicable.

Data Availability Statement: Not applicable.

Conflicts of Interest: The authors declare no conflict of interest.

References

1. Giansanti, D.; Pochini, M.; Giovagnoli, M.R. Integration of Tablet Technologies in the e-Laboratory of Cytology: A Health Technology Assessment. *Telemed. e-Health* **2014**, *20*, 909–915. [CrossRef]
2. Giansanti, D.; Pochini, M.; Giovagnoli, M.R. How Tablet Technology Is Going to Change Cooperative Diagnosis in the Cytology e-Laboratory. *Telemed. e-Health* **2013**, *19*, 991–993. [CrossRef]
3. Giansanti, D.; Grigioni, M.; D'Avenio, G.; Morelli, S.; Maccioni, G.; Bondi, A.; Giovagnoli, M.R. Virtual microscopy and digital cytology: State of the art. *Annali dell'Istituto Superiore Sanità* **2010**, *46*, 115–122.
4. Giansanti, D.; Castrichella, L.; Giovagnoli, M.R. Telepathology Requires Specific Training for the Technician in the Biomedical Laboratory. *Telemed. e-Health* **2008**, *14*, 801–807. [CrossRef] [PubMed]
5. Giansanti, D.; Castrichella, L.; Giovagnoli, M.R. The Design of a Health Technology Assessment System in Telepathology. *Telemed. e-Health* **2008**, *14*, 570–575. [CrossRef] [PubMed]

6. Avanzo, M.; Trianni, A.; Botta, F.; Talamonti, C.; Stasi, M.; Iori, M. Artificial Intelligence and the Medical Physicist: Welcome to the Machine. *Appl. Sci.* **2021**, *11*, 1691. [CrossRef]
7. Boschetto, A.; Pochini, M.; Bottini, L.; Giovagnoli, M.; Giansanti, D. The focus emulation and image enhancement in digital cytology: An experience using the software Mathematica. *Comput. Methods Biomech. Biomed. Eng. Imaging Vis.* **2014**, *3*, 1–7. [CrossRef]
8. Available online: https://www.virtualpathology.leeds.ac.uk/ (accessed on 6 July 2021).
9. Available online: https://www.virtualpathology.leeds.ac.uk/slides/library/ (accessed on 6 July 2021).
10. Available online: https://www.virtualpathology.leeds.ac.uk/slides/library/view.php?path=%2FResearch_4%2FTeaching%2FEducation%2FManchester_FRCPath%2FDN%2F124388.svs. (accessed on 6 July 2021).
11. Available online: http://dicom.nema.org/Dicom (accessed on 6 July 2021).
12. Available online: http://dicom.nema.org/Dicom/DICOMWSI/ (accessed on 6 July 2021).
13. Latonen, L.; Ruusuvuori, P. Building a central repository landmarks a new era for artificial intelligence–assisted digital pathology development in Europe. *Eur. J. Cancer* **2021**, *150*, 31–32. [CrossRef]
14. Aeffner, F.; Sing, T.; Turner, O.C. Special Issue on Digital Pathology, Tissue Image Analysis, Artificial Intelligence, and Machine Learning: Approximation of the Effect of Novel Technologies on Toxicologic Pathology. *Toxicol. Pathol.* **2021**, *49*, 705–708. [CrossRef] [PubMed]
15. Sobhani, F.; Robinson, R.; Hamidinekoo, A.; Roxanis, I.; Somaiah, N.; Yuan, Y. Artificial intelligence and digital pathology: Opportunities and implications for immuno-oncology. *Biochim. Biophys. Acta Rev. Cancer* **2021**, *1875*, 188520. [CrossRef] [PubMed]
16. Abdolahi, M.; Salehi, M.; Shokatian, I.; Reiazi, R. Artificial intelligence in automatic classification of invasive ductal carcinoma breast cancer in digital pathology images. *Med. J. Islam. Repub. Iran* **2020**, *34*, 965–973. [CrossRef]
17. Sakamoto, T.; Furukawa, T.; Lami, K.; Pham, H.H.N.; Uegami, W.; Kuroda, K.; Kawai, M.; Sakanashi, H.; Cooper, L.A.D.; Bychkov, A.; et al. A narrative review of digital pathology and artificial intelligence: Focusing on lung cancer. *Transl. Lung Cancer Res.* **2020**, *9*, 2255–2276. [CrossRef] [PubMed]
18. Bera, K.; Katz, I.; Madabhushi, A. Reimagining T Staging Through Artificial Intelligence and Machine Learning Image Processing Approaches in Digital Pathology. *JCO Clin. Cancer Inform.* **2020**, *4*, 1039–1050. [CrossRef] [PubMed]
19. Salama, M.E.; Macon, W.R.; Pantanowitz, L. Is the time right to start using digital pathology and artificial intelligence for the diagnosis of lymphoma? *J. Pathol. Inform.* **2020**, *11*. [CrossRef] [PubMed]
20. Browning, L.; Colling, R.; Rakha, E.; Rajpoot, N.; Rittscher, J.; James, J.A.; Salto-Tellez, M.; Snead, D.R.J.; Verrill, C. Digital pathology and artificial intelligence will be key to supporting clinical and academic cellular pathology through COVID-19 and future crises: The PathLAKE consortium perspective. *J. Clin. Pathol.* **2021**, *74*, 443–447. [CrossRef] [PubMed]
21. Parwani, A.V.; Amin, M.B. Convergence of Digital Pathology and Artificial Intelligence Tools in Anatomic Pathology Practice: Current Landscape and Future Directions. *Adv. Anat. Pathol.* **2020**, *27*, 221–226. [CrossRef]
22. Harmon, S.A.; Sanford, T.H.; Brown, G.T.; Yang, C.; Mehralivand, S.; Jacob, J.M.; Valera, V.A.; Shih, J.H.; Agarwal, P.K.; Choyke, P.L.; et al. Multiresolution Application of Artificial Intelligence in Digital Pathology for Prediction of Positive Lymph Nodes From Primary Tumors in Bladder Cancer. *JCO Clin. Cancer Inform.* **2020**, *4*, 367–382. [CrossRef] [PubMed]
23. Parwani, A.V. Next generation diagnostic pathology: Use of digital pathology and artificial intelligence tools to augment a pathological diagnosis. *Diagn. Pathol.* **2019**, *14*, 1–3. [CrossRef] [PubMed]
24. Turner, O.C.; Aeffner, F.; Bangari, D.S.; High, W.; Knight, B.; Forest, T.; Cossic, B.; Himmel, L.E.; Rudmann, D.G.; Bawa, B.; et al. Society of Toxicologic Pathology Digital Pathology and Image Analysis Special Interest Group Article*: Opinion on the Application of Artificial Intelligence and Machine Learning to Digital Toxicologic Pathology. *Toxicol. Pathol.* **2020**, *48*, 277–294. [CrossRef] [PubMed]
25. Bera, K.; Schalper, K.A.; Rimm, D.L.; Velcheti, V.; Madabhushi, A. Artificial intelligence in digital pathology—New tools for diagnosis and precision oncology. *Nat. Rev. Clin. Oncol.* **2019**, *16*, 703–715. [CrossRef] [PubMed]
26. Colling, R.; Pitman, H.; Oien, K.; Rajpoot, N.; Macklin, P.S.; CM-Path AI in Histopathology Working Group; Snead, D.; Sackville, T.; Verrill, C. Artificial intelligence in digital pathology: A roadmap to routine use in clinical practice. *J. Pathol.* **2019**, *249*, 143–150. [CrossRef]
27. Niazi, M.K.K.; Parwani, A.V.; Gurcan, M.N. Digital pathology and artificial intelligence. *Lancet Oncol.* **2019**, *20*, e253–e261. [CrossRef]
28. Tizhoosh, H.R.; Pantanowitz, L. Artificial intelligence and digital pathology: Challenges and opportunities. *J. Pathol. Inform.* **2018**, *9*, 38. [CrossRef] [PubMed]
29. Avanzo, M.; Pirrone, G.; Mileto, M.; Massarut, S.; Stancanello, J.; Baradaran-Ghahfarokhi, M.; Rink, A.; Barresi, L.; Vinante, L.; Piccoli, C.; et al. Prediction of skin dose in low-kV intraoperative radiotherapy using machine learning models trained on results of in vivo dosimetry. *Med. Phys.* **2019**, *46*, 1447–1454. [CrossRef] [PubMed]
30. Available online: https://pubmed.ncbi.nlm.nih.gov/?term=%28digital+pathology+%5BTitle%5D%29+AND+%28deep+learning+%5BTitle%5D%29&sort=date&size=200 (accessed on 6 July 2021).
31. Available online: https://pubmed.ncbi.nlm.nih.gov/?term=%28digital+pathology+%5BTitle%5D%29+AND+%28machine+learning+%5BTitle%5D%29&sort=date&size=200 (accessed on 6 July 2021).

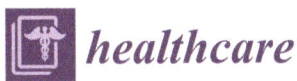

Article

Artificial Intelligence in Digital Pathology: What Is the Future? Part 2: *An Investigation on the Insiders*

Maria Rosaria Giovagnoli [1], Sara Ciucciarelli [1], Livia Castrichella [1] and Daniele Giansanti [2,*]

[1] Facoltà di Medicina e Psicologia, Università Sapienza Roma, Piazzale Aldo Moro, 00185 Rome, Italy; mr.giovagnoli.univ.sap@hotmail.com (M.R.G.); s.ciucciarelli.univ.sap@hotmail.com (S.C.); l.castrichella.univ.sap@hotmail.com (L.C.)

[2] Centre Tisp, Istituto Superiore di Sanità, 00161 Rome, Italy

* Correspondence: daniele.giansanti@iss.it; Tel.: +39-06-49902701

Abstract: *Motivation:* This study deals with the introduction of artificial intelligence (AI) in digital pathology (DP). The study starts from the highlights of a companion paper. *Objective:* The aim was to investigate the consensus and acceptance of the insiders on this issue. *Procedure:* An electronic survey based on the standardized package Microsoft Forms (Microsoft, Redmond, WA, USA) was proposed to a sample of biomedical laboratory technicians (149 admitted in the study, 76 males, 73 females, mean age 44.2 years). *Results:* The survey showed no criticality. It highlighted (a) the good perception of the basic training on both groups, and (b) a uniformly low perceived knowledge of AI (as arisen from the graded questions). Expectations, perceived general impact, perceived changes in the *work-flow*, and worries clearly emerged in the study. *Conclusions:* The of AI in DP is an unstoppable process, as well as the increase of the digitalization in the *health domain*. Stakeholders must not look with suspicion towards AI, which can represent an important resource, but should invest in monitoring and consensus training initiatives based also on electronic surveys.

Keywords: e-health; medical devices; m-health; digital-pathology; picture archive and communication system; artificial intelligence; cytology; histology; diagnostic pathology

1. Introduction

In a complementary study [1] we dealt with the introduction of artificial intelligence (AI) in digital pathology (DP). This could lead to a *second revolution* in pathological diagnostics (starting from the *first revolution* determined by the introduction of DP techniques both in *eHealth* and *mHealth* [2,3]). Most AI applications [1] take place in diagnostic imaging. However, there are many important implications related to the introduction of AI. These implications involve *other disciplines* (not only connected to imaging) and *other activities*, from the *work-flow* to the training. In our study [1] we recalled the passages that led to the first revolution of diagnostic pathology, represented by DP. We dedicated particular attention to the critical issues, given that AI will rely heavily on it. In the same study, we highlighted the opportunities and the challenges of AI according to the most recent studies [4–20]. Some important development guidelines have been identified. The DP developments with AI have been identified [20]. AI shows in DP (A) the potentiality to access and correlate large amount of data, and (B) direct prospective in the world of diagnostics.

Regarding *A*, both radiological and pathology images are stored in the *picture archiving and communication systems* (PACs). Moreover, with the introduction of electronic health records (EHRs), systematic collections of patient health information have been made available. They include qualitative data, medical records, and laboratory and diagnostics information. AI, if applied to these large digital stores, could prove useful for epidemiological, clinical, and research studies.

Regarding *B*, two aspects are emerging:

- The development of the DP, due to the introduction of *whole-slide scanners* and the *progress of computer vision algorithms*, have significantly grown the usage of AI. It can perform tumor diagnosis, subtyping, grading, staging, and prognostic prediction
- The pathological diagnosis of the future could merge proteomics and genomics in the BIG-DATA.

The challenges to tackle and the evident opportunities of AI in DP were recently categorized in [19]. These challenges were therefore recalled in [1], starting from the grid identified in [19]. The following transversal issues to be considered in these challenges were introduced and discussed [1]:

1. Delay of digital cytology.
2. Greater complexity in the introduction of AI in digital cytology.
3. Focus on the DICOM WSI standard.
4. Attention to both eHealth and mHealth.
5. New training models must adapt to AI in DP.
6. Need for standardization actions.
7. Extensive acceptance surveys on professionals.
8. Need to focus on all the professionals involved.

All that is highlighted in the above cross-cutting issues is of strong scientific interest. These issues are basic to plan a routine introduction of AI in DP.

We intend with this study to concentrate on some of the points detected.

We intend to propose a survey (*point 7*) focused on the professionals involved (*point 8*) to investigate the state of acceptance and the consensus on the introduction of AI in DP. Prior to this study, the experience reported in [21] focused on pathological diagnostics (*a single aspect of DP*), on a *single profession,* and proposed a non-validated and non-standardized questionnaire on the acceptance of AI in general. Despite limitations, several interesting findings were uncovered. Overall, respondents carried generally positive attitudes towards AI, excitement in AI as a diagnostic tool to facilitate improvements in *work-flow* efficiency, and quality assurance in pathology. Importantly, even within the most optimistic cohort, a significant number of respondents endorsed concerns about AI, including the potential for job displacement and replacement. Overall, around 80% of respondents predicted the introduction of AI technology in the pathology laboratory within the coming decade. The study focused on one single professional [21]; however, many other professionals are revolving around the introduction of AI in DP, ranging from the pathologist up to the biomedical laboratory technician.

There are many other aspects to be taken into consideration besides the diagnostic aspects [21]. We must consider, for example [1,19,20], the peculiarity of digital cytology and of digital histology, omics (e.g., genomics and proteomics), integration with BIGDATA, integration with historical and clinical data of the patient, the search for slide labelling, quality control, the integration of DP with digital radiology, training, risk analysis, therapy, and prevention.

The goal of our study was to

- Propose an electronic survey (based on a standardized software package) dedicated to the introduction of AI in DP, considering both the opportunities of AI in their entirety [1,19,20] (not limited to pathological diagnostics) and the involved professionals.
- Submit it electronically to a first sample of insiders.
- Analyze the outcome.

2. Materials and Methods

In line with the aim of the study, we decided to propose a survey to investigate the acceptance and the consensus of the insiders. Preliminarily, we addressed the aspects of privacy and data security. The questionnaire was checked for the compliance to the European GDPR 679/2016 and the Italian Decree 101/2018, as required by the Data Protection Offices. The questionnaire was planned as anonymous. The topic did not concern clinical trials on humans, but only opinions and expressions of their thoughts. In consideration of this, it was not considered necessary to proceed with the formal approval procedures from the Institutional Review Board (see footnote at the end). The standard Microsoft Forms package (Microsoft Forms, Redmond, WA, USA) was chosen.

This package is also available with a free Microsoft account (live, outlook, or hotmail, for example), but in this case, it has important limitations (for example, the maximum number of participants is limited to 200). The data acquired by means of Microsoft Forms represent a public register from a legal point of view. Therefore, data need to be strongly protected by means of a strong cybersecurity approach. This is not feasible using only a free Microsoft account.

Companies that have centrally installed the Microsoft 365 App Business Premium suite have Microsoft Forms available to their users with greater potential than the free version (for example, the maximum limit of participants is raised to 50,000). All users can have access through their own domain account guaranteed by the corporate cybersecurity standards (which must comply with the international regulations in force) supported by network and system security tools and policies managed by the company. Specific checks are possible on the IPs (registering, for example, the duplicate access for further dataprocess). Data are therefore protected by the corporate cybersecurity systems, guaranteeing (at least from the system point of view) the inviolability of the data. In consideration of this, we have decided to use the software Microsoft Forms, provided through the Microsoft 365 Business Premium suite, to design an electronic survey. It is the tool recommended by the company's DPO. It should be noted that if a tool other than those available in this suite (e.g., Google forms or Survey Monkey) had been used, the DPO would have requested a specific report and a cybersecurity audit. The authorization to use it would not have been guaranteed. The use of both an internally recommended tool (respecting the cybersecurity) and the plan to submit the electronic survey (eS) anonymously simplified the authorization process. However, we decided to maintain the database as a register, respecting the security criteria identified by the company rules in accordance with the law. The procedure used in the design and submission of the survey adhered to the *SURGE Checklist* [22].

We decided to submit the survey to the key professionals and therefore disseminated it through social media, such as Facebook, LinkedIn, Twitter, Instagram, WhatsApp, Association Sites, and in general, following a *peer-to-peer* dissemination. We submitted the survey to biomedical laboratory technicians during their course of study (*BLT-DCS*) and after the course of the study (*BLT-ACS*). The interactive survey is available in [23]. A print can also be found in [24].

Two questions (N.2 and N.3) stratify by age and sex [23,24]. Two initial questions (N.4 and N.5) categorize the sample on the basis of the training background. In consideration of the objective of this study and the survey, we also managed the survey as a virtual focus group, with careful considerations to the consensus issues related to all the aspects of the introduction of AI in DP [1,19,20]. We started from the training up to the relationships and integration with omics, BIG-DATA, and digital radiology. The methodological approach primarily involves submitting both to *BLT-DCS* and *BLT-ACS* surveys. Figure 1 shows the CONSORT diagram. The final records were 211 in number. Two records were excluded because the answers to the open questions were not coherent.

The subjects passing the requirements for the inclusion according to the selection criteria (*BLT-DCS* or *BLT-ACS*) were 149 (Table 1).

The quantitative variables depended on subjective answers based on qualitative perceptions (see for example in the following the graded questions or the modules in the Likert scale). The survey used *open question, choice question, multiple choice questions, Likert questions,* and *graded questions.*

We established a six-level psychometric scale for the *Likert scale* and the *graded questions*. It was possible therefore to assign a minimum score of one and a maximum of six with a *theoretical mean value* (TMV) of 3.5. We can refer to the TMV for comparison in the analysis of the answers. An average value of the answers below TMV indicates a more negative than positive response. An average value above TMV indicates a more positive than negative response.

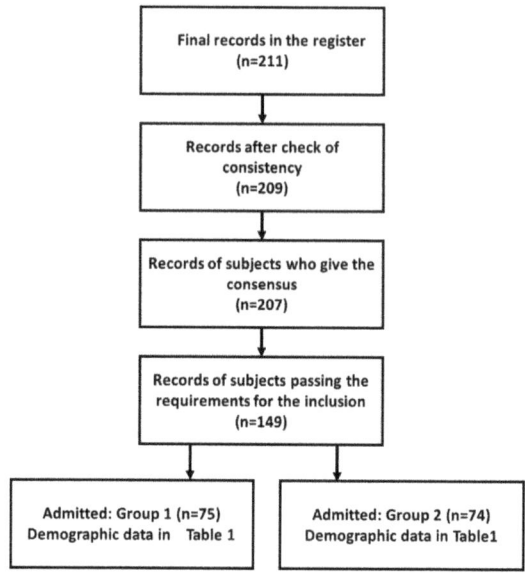

Figure 1. The CONSORT diagram.

Table 1. Characteristics of the admitted to the study the DCS and the ACS.

Submission	Participants	Males/Females	Min Age/Max Age	Mean Age
Biomedical laboratory technicians under the course of the study (BLT-DCS)	75	39/36	21/36	25.3
Biomedical laboratory technicians after the course of the study (BLT-ACS)	74	37/37	25/59	41.8

The trend of each one of these variables, estimated by an average value, can move in both the two directions, toward the higher score of 6 or toward the lower score of 1, suggesting for a two-tailed test. For the variables related to the *multiple-choice* questions, we planned a frequency analysis.

For the verification of data normality, we used the Shapiro–Wilk test that is preferable for small samples such as ours.

We applied Student's t-test (with a p-value <0.01 for the significance of the difference), when comparing the values between the two groups.

We applied the χ^2 test (with a p-value <0.01 for the significance) in the frequency analysis. The software SPSS Statistics version V.24 was used in the study.

The Cohen's d effect size was estimated to be 0.498. Samples with $N > 60$ were estimated suitable to the study.

We established a six-level psychometric scale in the graded questions and in the Likert scale.

The survey was proposed from 1 June 2021 until 23 August 2021.

3. Results

Table 2 shows the answers to the graded *questions*. Both questions Q6 and Q7, not focused directly on AI, received an average response value above the TMV threshold.

Table 2. Answers for the graded questions.

Feature	Rating DCS	Rating ACS	*p*-Value
Q6: Degree of knowledge in computer science	4.8	4.9	0.009
Q7: Degree of knowledge of biomedical technologies	4.7	4.7	0.134
Q9: Degree of knowledge of AI (in general)	3.3	3.1	0.009
Q10: Degree of knowledge of AI (in biomedical sector)	3.4	3.2	0.009
Q11: Degree of direct knowledge of technologies and applications of AI (in biomedical sector)	1.8	1.3	0.008

However, Q6 showed a significantly higher value in the student group (*p*-value < 0.01), while Q7 showed a consistent value between the two groups (*p*-value = 0.134 >> 0.01).

The responses related to AI, Q8–10, showed a value below the current TMV threshold in the two groups (*p*-value < 0.01).

Tables 3 and 4 highlight the outcomes for the two Likert scales in detail. In the first Likert scale (Table 3), *imaging* (cytological and histological) received the highest score for the two groups, followed by applications in *omics and quality control*. Table 4 shows the significant highest values for the first group in the second Likert scale dedicated to other sectors of applications.

Table 3. Detailed answers in the Likert scale to the question of "In which specific sectors of biomedical diagnostics do you think the introduction of artificial intelligence is most promising?".

Feature	Rating DCS	Rating ACS	*p*-Value
Digital cytology	4.9	4.5	0.008
Digital histology	4.8	4.4	0.009
Omics (e.g., genomics and proteomics)	4.6	4.3	0.008
Integration with BIG-DATA	3.9	3.7	0.008
Integration with historical and clinical data of the patient	4.1	3.8	0.009
Search for slide labeling	3.9	3.6	0.009
Quality control	4.1	3.8	0.009
Integration of DP with digital radiology	4.2	3.9	0.009
Quality control	4.5	4.2	0.008
Integration with the virtual medical record	3.9	3.7	0.008
Training	3.9	3.6	0.008

Table 4. Detailed answers in the Likert scale to the question of "In which more general sectors do you think artificial intelligence is useful?".

Feature	Rating DCS	Rating ACS	p-Value
Risk analysis	4.3	3.7	0.008
Therapy	4.4	3.8	0.008
Prevention	3.9	3.6	0.009

The *multiple-choice questions* are useful for obtaining strategic information, for example, for scientific societies or consensus activities. We decided to proceed as follows, in consideration of the peculiarity of these modules. We analyzed the two samples joined into one sample and performed a statistical approach based on a frequency analysis, using the test described in the methods.

For question Q13 *"I think artificial intelligence in my field"*, the two most popular statements were *"It will be useful but complementary"* number of votes = 83 and *"It will not catch on"* number of votes = 78 (p-value = 0.008).

For question Q14 *"How can I be of use to AI in my filed"*, the two most popular statements were *"In performance monitoring"* number of votes = 90 and *"As an operational manager of its use"* number of votes = 81 (p-value = 0.008).

For question Q15 *"How will AI help me"*, the two most popular statements were *"Increased automatism"* number of votes = 79 and *"Reduction of physical fatigue"* number of votes = 61 (p-value = 0.009).

4. Discussion and Conclusions

The use of AI is increasingly spreading in many medical sectors.

A particularly important area for applications is that of images. A simple search on PubMed with the key

(artificial intelligence [Title/Abstract]) AND (image [Title/Abstract])

shows 2290 results as of 23 August 2021 (907 in 2021).

This justifies the need of focusing on studies of acceptance, in consideration of both the interest of the scholars and the possible opportunities in the clinical routine.

Some studies are also demonstrating the importance of AI tools, not only in imaging, but also in other applications where *data mining from large volumes of data must be applied*.

For example, the study reported in [25] showed how AI is useful for determining cardiovascular risk in athletes through *data mining of distributed databases*.

The COVID-19 pandemic has also highlighted *the broad-spectrum potential of AI*. In a recent review [26], for example, relevant papers were selected that address the adoption of artificial intelligence and new technologies in the management of pandemics and communicable diseases such as SARS-CoV-2.

These studies focused on environmental measures; acquisition and sharing of knowledge in the general population and among clinicians; development and management of drugs and vaccines; remote psychological support of patients; remote monitoring, diagnosis, and follow-up; and maximization and rationalization of human and material resources in the hospital environment. The study described in [27] showed that *AI-based scores with a purely data-driven selection of features* are feasible and effective for the prediction of mortality among patients with COVID-19 pneumonia.

The three illustrated potentials [25–27] are also important in DP. In fact, in DP, the need for categorizing images merges with the need to make decisions and/or deduce approaches through actions on large databases and data sets or with other needs not based on medical images [1,19,20]. The implications are multifaceted. It is necessary to carry out direct studies on the opinion of insiders in view of the introduction of the clinical routine of AI.

Therefore, the need and the justification of studies such as ours that tackle the introduction of AI focusing on acceptance and with a broad approach clearly emerges from these articles [25–27].

Very few studies have begun to address the insiders' opinion on the introduction of AI in DP. By searching in PubMed with the key

((digital pathology [Title/Abstract]) AND (artificial intelligence [Title/Abstract])) AND (survey [Title/Abstract])-even with alternative terms to the survey-

we found as of 23 August 2021 only two studies based on non-validated and non-standardized questionnaires.

The first study [28] was conducted at a scientific meeting (the 14th Banff Conference). Since the meeting, a survey with international participation of mostly pathologists (81%) was conducted, showing that whole slide imaging is available at the majority of centers (71%), but that artificial intelligence (AI)/machine learning was only used in ≈12% of centers, with a wide variety of programs/algorithms employed.

The second study [29] reports the results of the Japanese questionnaire survey conducted in 2008–2009 on telepathology and virtual slide. Moreover, in addition to the questionnaire, the effectiveness of an experimental automatic pathology diagnostic aid system using computer artificial intelligence was investigated by checking its rate of correct diagnosis for given prostate carcinoma digital images.

This demonstrates the importance of focusing on wide-ranging survey studies in this field. From this research, it clearly emerges that specific studies, such as ours based on wide range questionnaires, have not been addressed until now. In fact, in the literature, there are currently only studies that deal with the topic only partially or secondarily [28,29].

This study was necessary to prepare a first survey dedicated to the acceptance of AI in DP focused on the insiders [1]. We submitted the survey on the professionals involved in the field. Many professionals are involved in the introduction of AI in DP, ranging from the bioengineer to the pathologist up to the biomedical laboratory technician. There is also no doubt that AI could represent a serious opportunity for the DP laboratories [5–18]. It is, however, the time to investigate the full introduction in the routine. The proposed study, for example, can be useful in view of consensus studies on the introduction of methods based on AI in DP in routine practices [1,19]. We have proposed a survey focused on these professionals that is, in an automatic manner, capable of electronically collecting their opinion and works as a structured virtual focus group.

The intent of this study was to carry out a first submission and to verify any criticalities in view of a wider use. There were no critical issues and the submission made it possible to collect information on a first sample of biomedical laboratory technicians in the training phase and subsequent phase.

A good perception of the basic training on both groups (albeit with a different score) and a uniformly low perceived knowledge of the use of AI emerged from the graded questions.

The *two Likert scales* made it possible to identify in a structured way, for the two groups, the wishes related to the use of AI in the medical field.

The *multiple-choice* questions, evaluated for the whole combined sample, allowed us to evaluate the perceived impact of AI in one's sector, the expectations towards AI, and the operational role towards AI. From a general point of view, the study presents three added values.

The *first added* value is [23,24] represented by the electronic tool with a wide range of aspects related to the use of AI in DP, having a direct impact on the *work-flow* and *job description* of the insiders.

The *second added* value is a contribution directed to respond to the need to tackle the challenges of the introduction of AI in DP. This product (after minimal changes) could be used by scientific and/or professional societies to monitor the evolution of the topic.

The *third added* value is represented by the outcome with reference to the two groups of *DCS* and *ACS* (promptly useful for the stakeholders).

From a general point of view, this article supports the initiatives that aim to facilitate the introduction of AI in a structured manner in DP. Future developments of the study foresee the enlargement of the submission to other professionals and a standardization for the scientific societies.

5. Limitations

This study represents a first step to investigate the acceptance and consensus on AI of insiders in the various applications and implications of DP. It was applied to a first professional and a first group of subjects. Future developments will have to include a broader submission involving other professionals, together with a review action by the scientific societies, in order to improve acceptance by the parties involved.

Author Contributions: Conceptualization, D.G. and M.R.G.; methodology, D.G. and L.C.; software, D.G. and S.C.; validation, D.G., M.R.G., and L.C.; formal analysis, all authors; investigation, all authors; resources, all authors; data curation, D.G.; writing—original draft preparation, D.G. and S.C.; writing—review and editing, D.G.; visualization, all authors; supervision, all authors; project administration, all authors; funding acquisition, none. All authors have read and agreed to the published version of the manuscript.

Funding: This research received no external funding.

Institutional Review Board Statement: Not applicable.

Informed Consent Statement: Not applicable.

Data Availability Statement: Not applicable.

Conflicts of Interest: The authors declare no conflict of interest.

References

1. Giovagnoli, M.; Giansanti, D. Artificial Intelligence in Digital Pathology: What Is the Future? *Part 1: From the Digital Slide Onwards*. *Healthcare* **2021**, *9*, 858. [CrossRef] [PubMed]
2. Giansanti, D.; Pochini, M.; Giovagnoli, M.R. Integration of Tablet Technologies in the e-Laboratory of Cytology: A Health Technology Assessment. *Telemed. e-Health* **2014**, *20*, 909–915. [CrossRef] [PubMed]
3. Giansanti, D.; Castrichella, L.; Giovagnoli, M.R. The Design of a Health Technology Assessment System in Telepathology. *Telemed. e-Health* **2008**, *14*, 570–575. [CrossRef] [PubMed]
4. Latonen, L.; Ruusuvuori, P. Building a central repository landmarks a new era for artificial intelligence–assisted digital pathology development in Europe. *Eur. J. Cancer* **2021**, *150*, 31–32. [CrossRef] [PubMed]
5. Aeffner, F.; Sing, T.; Turner, O.C. Special Issue on Digital Pathology, Tissue Image Analysis, Artificial Intelligence, and Machine Learning: Approximation of the Effect of Novel Technologies on Toxicologic Pathology. *Toxicol. Pathol.* **2021**, *49*, 705–708. [CrossRef]
6. Sobhani, F.; Robinson, R.; Hamidinekoo, A.; Roxanis, I.; Somaiah, N.; Yuan, Y. Artificial intelligence and digital pathology: Opportunities and implications for immuno-oncology. *Biochim. Biophys. Acta (BBA) Bioenerg.* **2021**, *1875*, 188520. [CrossRef]
7. Abdolahi, M.; Salehi, M.; Shokatian, I.; Reiazi, R. Artificial intelligence in automatic classification of invasive ductal carcinoma breast cancer in digital pathology images. *Med. J. Islam. Repub. Iran* **2020**, *34*, 965–973. [CrossRef]
8. Sakamoto, T.; Furukawa, T.; Lami, K.; Pham, H.H.N.; Uegami, W.; Kuroda, K.; Kawai, M.; Sakanashi, H.; Cooper, L.A.D.; Bychkov, A.; et al. A narrative review of digital pathology and artificial intelligence: Focusing on lung cancer. *Transl. Lung Cancer Res.* **2020**, *9*, 2255–2276. [CrossRef]
9. Bera, K.; Katz, I.; Madabhushi, A. Reimagining T Staging Through Artificial Intelligence and Machine Learning Image Processing Approaches in Digital Pathology. *JCO Clin. Cancer Inform.* **2020**, *4*, 1039–1050. [CrossRef] [PubMed]
10. Salama, M.E.; Macon, W.R.; Pantanowitz, L. Is the time right to start using digital pathology and artificial intelligence for the diagnosis of lymphoma? *J. Pathol. Inform.* **2020**, *11*, 16. [CrossRef]
11. Browning, L.; Colling, R.; Rakha, E.; Rajpoot, N.; Rittscher, J.; James, J.A.; Salto-Tellez, M.; Snead, D.R.J.; Verrill, C. Digital pathology and artificial intelligence will be key to supporting clinical and academic cellular pathology through COVID-19 and future crises: The PathLAKE consortium perspective. *J. Clin. Pathol.* **2020**, *74*, 443–447. [CrossRef]
12. Parwani, A.V.; Amin, M.B. Convergence of Digital Pathology and Artificial Intelligence Tools in Anatomic Pathology Practice: Current Landscape and Future Directions. *Adv. Anat. Pathol.* **2020**, *27*, 221–226. [CrossRef]
13. Harmon, S.A.; Sanford, T.H.; Brown, G.T.; Yang, C.; Mehralivand, S.; Jacob, J.M.; Valera, V.A.; Shih, J.H.; Agarwal, P.K.; Choyke, P.L.; et al. Multiresolution Application of Artificial Intelligence in Digital Pathology for Prediction of Positive Lymph Nodes From Primary Tumors in Bladder Cancer. *JCO Clin. Cancer Inform.* **2020**, *4*, 367–382. [CrossRef] [PubMed]

14. Parwani, A.V. Next generation diagnostic pathology: Use of digital pathology and artificial intelligence tools to augment a pathological diagnosis. *Diagn. Pathol.* **2019**, *14*, 1–3. [CrossRef] [PubMed]
15. Turner, O.C.; Aeffner, F.; Bangari, D.S.; High, W.; Knight, B.; Forest, T.; Cossic, B.; Himmel, L.E.; Rudmann, D.G.; Bawa, B.; et al. Society of Toxicologic Pathology Digital Pathology and Image Analysis Special Interest Group Article*: Opinion on the Application of Artificial Intelligence and Machine Learning to Digital Toxicologic Pathology. *Toxicol. Pathol.* **2019**, *48*, 277–294. [CrossRef]
16. Bera, K.; Schalper, K.A.; Rimm, D.L.; Velcheti, V.; Madabhushi, A. Artificial intelligence in digital pathology—New tools for diagnosis and precision oncology. *Nat. Rev. Clin. Oncol.* **2019**, *16*, 703–715. [CrossRef] [PubMed]
17. Colling, R.; Pitman, H.; Oien, K.; Rajpoot, N.; Macklin, P.; CM-Path AI in Histopathology Working Group; Snead, D.; Sackville, T.; Verrill, C. Artificial intelligence in digital pathology: A roadmap to routine use in clinical practice. *J. Pathol.* **2019**, *249*, 143–150. [CrossRef] [PubMed]
18. Niazi, M.K.K.; Parwani, A.V.; Gurcan, M.N. Digital pathology and artificial intelligence. *Lancet Oncol.* **2019**, *20*, e253–e261. [CrossRef]
19. Tizhoosh, H.R.; Pantanowitz, L. Artificial intelligence and digital pathology: Challenges and opportunities. *J. Pathol. Inform.* **2018**, *9*, 38. [CrossRef]
20. Avanzo, M.; Trianni, A.; Botta, F.; Talamonti, C.; Stasi, M.; Iori, M. Artificial Intelligence and the Medical Physicist: Welcome to the Machine. *Appl. Sci.* **2021**, *11*, 1691. [CrossRef]
21. Sarwar, S.; Dent, A.; Faust, K.; Richer, M.; Djuric, U.; Van Ommeren, R.; Diamandis, P. Physician perspectives on integration of artificial intelligence into diagnostic pathology. *NPJ Digit. Med.* **2019**, *2*, 1–7. [CrossRef] [PubMed]
22. Grimshaw, J. SURGE (The SUrvey Reporting GuidelinE). In *Guidelines for Reporting Health Research: A User's Manual*; John Wiley & Sons, Ltd.: Oxford, UK, 2014; pp. 206–213. [CrossRef]
23. Available online: https://forms.office.com/Pages/ResponsePage.aspx?id=_ccwzxZmYkutg7V0sn1ZEvPNtNci4kVMpoVUounzQ3tUNjNSVENQU01DRTVVWUkxMVg5V0tBQUhKMy4u (accessed on 9 October 2021).
24. Available online: https://drive.google.com/file/d/1Av6cNrjkOi-00VNT7vtqBEZeDWpKnZXP/view?usp=sharing (accessed on 9 October 2021).
25. Barbieri, D.; Chawla, N.; Zaccagni, L.; Grgurinović, T.; Šarac, J.; Čoklo, M.; Missoni, S. Predicting Cardiovascular Risk in Athletes: Resampling Improves Classification Performance. *Int. J. Environ. Res. Public Health* **2020**, *17*, 7923. [CrossRef] [PubMed]
26. Barbieri, D.; Giuliani, E.; Del Prete, A.; Losi, A.; Villani, M.; Barbieri, A. How Artificial Intelligence and New Technologies Can Help the Management of the COVID-19 Pandemic. *Int. J. Environ. Res. Public Health* **2021**, *18*, 7648. [CrossRef] [PubMed]
27. Halasz, G.; Sperti, M.; Villani, M.; Michelucci, U.; Agostoni, P.; Biagi, A.; Rossi, L.; Botti, A.; Mari, C.; Maccarini, M.; et al. A Machine Learning Approach for Mortality Prediction in COVID-19 Pneumonia: Development and Evaluation of the Piacenza Score. *J. Med. Internet Res.* **2021**, *23*, e29058. [CrossRef] [PubMed]
28. Farris, A.B.; Moghe, I.; Wu, S.; Hogan, J.; Cornell, L.D.; Alexander, M.P.; Kers, J.; Demetris, A.J.; Levenson, R.M.; Tomaszewski, J.; et al. Banff Digital Pathology Working Group: Going digital in transplant pathology. *Am. J. Transplant.* **2020**, *20*, 2392–2399. [CrossRef]
29. Tsuchihashi, Y. Expanding application of digital pathology in Japan—From education, telepathology to autodiagnosis. *Diagn. Pathol.* **2011**, *6*, S19. [CrossRef]

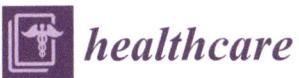

Review

Artificial Intelligence Advances in the World of Cardiovascular Imaging

Bhakti Patel [1] and Amgad N. Makaryus [1,2,3,*]

1. Donald and Barbara Zucker School of Medicine at Hofstra/Northwell, Hofstra University, Hempstead, NY 11549, USA; bpatel10@pride.hofstra.edu
2. Department of Cardiology, Nassau University Medical Center, East Meadow, NY 11554, USA
3. Department of Cardiology, Northwell Health, Manhasset, NY 11030, USA
* Correspondence: amakaryus@numc.edu

Abstract: The tremendous advances in digital information and communication technology have entered everything from our daily lives to the most intricate aspects of medical and surgical care. These advances are seen in electronic and mobile health and allow many new applications to further improve and make the diagnoses of patient diseases and conditions more precise. In the area of digital radiology with respect to diagnostics, the use of advanced imaging tools and techniques is now at the center of evaluation and treatment. Digital acquisition and analysis are central to diagnostic capabilities, especially in the field of cardiovascular imaging. Furthermore, the introduction of artificial intelligence (AI) into the world of digital cardiovascular imaging greatly broadens the capabilities of the field both with respect to advancement as well as with respect to complete and accurate diagnosis of cardiovascular conditions. The application of AI in recognition, diagnostics, protocol automation, and quality control for the analysis of cardiovascular imaging modalities such as echocardiography, nuclear cardiac imaging, cardiovascular computed tomography, cardiovascular magnetic resonance imaging, and other imaging, is a major advance that is improving rapidly and continuously. We document the innovations in the field of cardiovascular imaging that have been brought about by the acceptance and implementation of AI in relation to healthcare professionals and patients in the cardiovascular field.

Keywords: artificial intelligence; information technology; cardiology; radiology; imaging

Citation: Patel, B.; Makaryus, A.N. Artificial Intelligence Advances in the World of Cardiovascular Imaging. *Healthcare* **2022**, *10*, 154. https://doi.org/10.3390/healthcare10010154

Academic Editors: Daniele Giansanti and Norbert Hosten

Received: 19 November 2021
Accepted: 11 January 2022
Published: 14 January 2022

Publisher's Note: MDPI stays neutral with regard to jurisdictional claims in published maps and institutional affiliations.

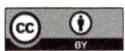

Copyright: © 2022 by the authors. Licensee MDPI, Basel, Switzerland. This article is an open access article distributed under the terms and conditions of the Creative Commons Attribution (CC BY) license (https://creativecommons.org/licenses/by/4.0/).

1. Introduction

In this age of technology, there have been numerous inventions created to expand the boundaries of medical treatment and diagnosis beyond their current capabilities. Among the technological advancements, artificial intelligence (AI) serves as a means to improve various technologies already in practice. Specifically, within the medical field, AI provides greater accuracy to help guide a patient's course of treatment. Physicians are able to make clear initial decisions on how to treat patients presenting with specific symptoms. There is also a reduction in human error seen with the greater precision and automaticity capabilities of artificial intelligence. AI is beneficial for patients themselves as well by guiding patients to understand their symptoms through phone applications that detail whether patients need to go to the emergency room or their local doctor's office based on acuity. Furthermore, AI has been used to strengthen the cardiac imaging modalities such as echocardiography, nuclear cardiac imaging, cardiovascular computed tomography, and cardiovascular magnetic resonance imaging. While AI has shown promise, limitations of AI include a lack of standardization and reproducibility of results as well as decision making and selection bias.

Artificial intelligence refers to the all-encompassing ability of mathematical algorithms to train machines to mimic human intelligence. With the use of programmed algorithms, machines are able to complete tasks, execute decisions, and recognize images [1]. Within AI, machine learning is a subset (Figure 1) that identifies patterns among big datasets. It has the unique ability to automatically improve analysis over time with more usage of data and experience. Essentially, machine learning works by implementing algorithms to create a model from a sample dataset without directly programming the decisions needed to be made [2]. This is particularly useful in fields such as medicine where decisions are not predictable and vary in every individual patient. Machine learning provides the opportunity to handle complex data with the ability to become more accurate over time. Machine learning itself can be classified as supervised and unsupervised (Table 1). These two techniques are applied in different situations. Particularly, supervised learning refers to when models are trained to analyze algorithms based on reference data that have already been entered. Thus, as it works from a reference dataset and applies the same pattern to a new dataset, supervised learning is very accurate [3,4]. Unsupervised learning refers to finding patterns in data on its own without any given reference. This is advantageous in finding hidden patterns that have not already been identified [3,5]. Despite its advantages, machine learning has its limitations, especially apparent when applied to the field of medicine. Specifically, machine learning can lead to bias when it comes to analyzing the dataset. This is due to the way the algorithms are organized which is to become better with more exposure to previous datasets. Therefore, this decreases the variety of data that machines have to make information other than what was previously represented [6].

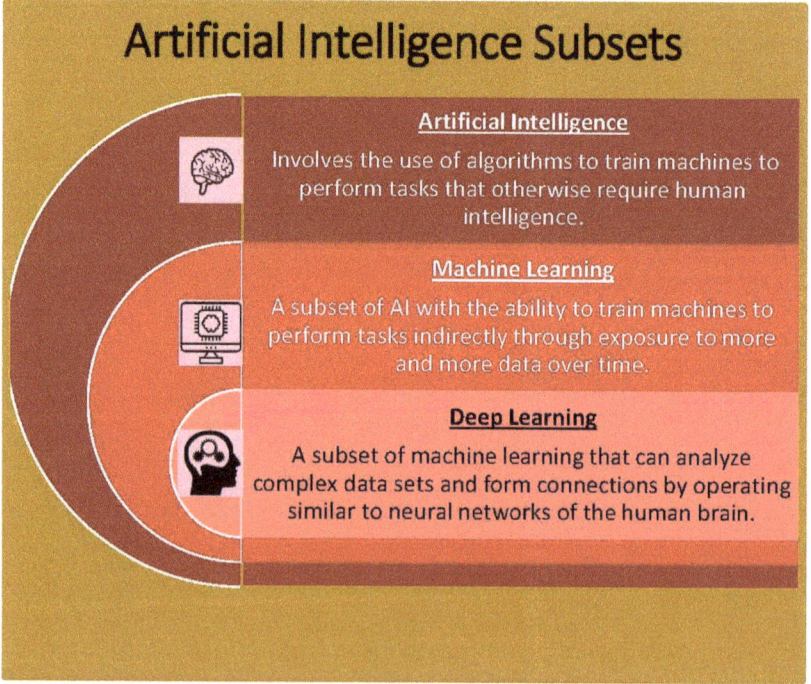

Figure 1. Artificial intelligence subsets into which the principles of AI can be divided.

Furthermore, deep learning is a subset of machine learning. Deep learning uses artificial neural networks to allow machines to train themselves in accomplishing tasks. In other words, it can discover complex relationships that cannot otherwise be analyzed simply by an equation. It works to inspect and analyze an unlimited number of inputs at the same time [7]. A deep convolutional neural network (DCNN) is a specific type of neural network that involves restricted connectivity. Specifically, DCNN is often used for classification tasks as well as detection and localization [8]. DCNNs operate by involving convolutional layers, where each layer combines information from neighboring inputs to have a larger field of view. This is beneficial to finding patterns like visual pieces within an image, such as shapes and lines [9].

Table 1. Methodology of supervised and unsupervised learning within machine learning.

Machine Learning Classification	Types of Problems Each Classification Is Used for
Supervised Learning—Uses reference data to analyze algorithms and apply the algorithms to a similar dataset [3]	**Classification**—Utilizes an algorithm to assign a dataset into specific categories. Specifically, draws conclusions on how specific categories in the dataset should be labeled. [4]
	Regression—Analyzes the relationship between dependent and independent variables, particularly for making projections [4]
Unsupervised Learning—Identifies hidden patterns in data without any given reference [3]	**Clustering**—Organizes unlabeled data based on similarities and differences [5]
	Dimension Reduction—Reduces the number of data inputs while preserving the data integrity; applied when there is an increased number of features or dimensions in a dataset [5]

Deep learning is beneficial over traditional machine learning as it requires less data for training and has more accuracy [10]. In particular, deep learning is most valuable with pattern recognition and image identification, particularly when working with large image datasets. Therefore, it is most effective for cardiovascular imaging, such as echocardiography, angiography, and cardiac magnetic resonance. This is especially true as deep learning has the ability to parse through insignificant or noisy data [1]. Although deep learning is useful with image recognition, it is limited insofar as its algorithm cannot be efficiently applied for all types of datasets. For example, simpler machine learning would be easier to use for datasets that are more defined and structured.

2. AI: General Medical Applications

The field of artificial intelligence allows for advancements to take place that expand the abilities of current technology. The goal of artificial intelligence is to create intelligence that has the ability for computers to solve problems and perform tasks, thus replicating the human mind [11]. AI involves the development of algorithms that can mimic the reasoning skills of humans in solving problems and deducing information in a methodical fashion. Over the years, AI has been applied to many different fields and used for a variety of purposes. Within medicine, AI has been used to improve diagnostic and treatment methods as well as efficiency with healthcare management [12]. For instance, most medical records are a collection of disorganized information hard to rifle through. However, with the application of AI, the information collected can allow physicians to understand a patient's complete medical information prior to making medical decisions in real time. Specifically, algorithms that allow for the ability to search for patients with significant family history or susceptibility of chronic diseases transform the usage of electronic medical records [13]. More efficiently organized electronic medical records ultimately serve as a tool for personalized medicine and early detection of diseases.

In addition to programming algorithms, AI has also been applied to physical objects, such as medical devices and robots. For example, robotic-assisted surgeries are more often utilized to operate on patients [14]. The quality of care is drastically improved with the use of robots in surgery as incisions are more minimally invasive. This allows for patients to experience less pain after the surgery and have a shorter recovery time. The robotic surgical tool also serves to dissect, cut, and suture in a more precise fashion. With the addition of AI, surgical robots can identify the movements and patterns of a surgeon performing an operation and convert these into actions for the robot to execute on its own [15]. Additionally, the use of robots eliminates human error from surgeons, such as with hand tremors or accidental cuts [16]. In fact, of the 17 million surgical procedures performed in the United States, it was found that there were 400,000 operations with adverse outcomes attributed to human error [17]. Furthermore, Rajih et al. found robotic surgery error on the da Vinci surgical system in 4.97% of 1228 cases evaluated between 2012 and 2015 [18]. In this case, the use of AI-led robots allows for benefits such as improving the quality of care and providing accuracy and stability to prevent more human error.

3. AI: Cardiology Imaging Applications

Machine learning is a branch of AI that is particularly useful in the interpretation of cardiovascular imaging because it can combine and correlate information from different sources for a physician to interpret efficiently [19]. Specifically, machine learning has the ability to use a variety of different approaches to analyze a greater quantity of information. Coronary artery disease (CAD) is one of the most prevalent cardiovascular disorders and is responsible for one in every five deaths [20]. Coronary artery disease is generally diagnosed with radionuclide myocardial perfusion imaging (MPI). With the addition of machine learning to supplement the MPI results, the patient-specific risk stratification is improved. A study by Seetharam et al. found evidence that machine learning is greater than parametric statistical models in predicting the presence of obstructive CAD, the need for revascularization, and potential adverse risks [21]. Specifically, Arsajani et al. conducted a study that evaluated the MPI device's accuracy of predicting CAD in 957 patients when used in adjunct with a learning algorithm compared to two experienced imaging readers. The results showed that the machine learning's sensitivity and specificity was significantly superior compared to the experienced readers [19]. Multiple cardiac imaging applications and pertinent publications relating to them (Table 2 and Figure 2) are detailed below and lead to generation of data that inform artificial intelligence algorithms to allow for analysis and evaluation.

Table 2. Pertinent publications regarding artificial intelligence.

Pertinent Publications Related to Artificial Intelligence in the Field of Cardiovascular Imaging	Findings in Publication
Improved accuracy of myocardial perfusion single-photon emission computed tomography [SPECT] for the detection of coronary artery disease using a support vector machine algorithm	Arsajani et al. found that the accuracy of predicting CAD with an MPI device improved significantly when in adjunct with a learning algorithm [22]
Fully Automated Echocardiogram Interpretation in Clinical Practice	Zhang et al. determined 96% accuracy in identifying images with echocardiography [22]
Machine learning of clinical variables and coronary artery calcium scoring for the prediction of obstructive coronary artery disease on coronary computed tomography angiography: analysis from the CONFIRM registry	Al'Aref et al.'s results showed a significantly more accurate assessment of obstructive CAD from CT imaging using machine learning with the coronary artery calcium score [21]
Cardiac Imaging on the Cusp of an Artificial Intelligence Revolution	Laser et al. determined that the right ventricle reconstruction with echocardiography and cardiac MRI had more accuracy compared to the gold standard direct cardiac MRI [23]

3.1. Echocardiography

Within the field of cardiology, AI has had a tremendous impact on how early and accurately patients are diagnosed as well as receive treatment. Echocardiography is a noninvasive diagnostic test that is performed on patients to detect or monitor the progression of cardiovascular diseases [17]. It is advantageous in visualizing the structure, function, and hemodynamics of the heart as well as any characteristic abnormalities. Specifically, echocardiography is beneficial as a cost-effective tool and can be performed at bedside rapidly with no known side effects [17]. On the other hand, a limitation of echocardiography is that it relies on a subjective interpretation of the images by the physician. Therefore, although obtaining the images is feasible with echocardiography, there is still a likelihood of an inaccurate diagnosis [23]. To address this limitation, AI provides the ability to produce accurate, consistent, and automated interpretations of echocardiograms [23]. Consequently, this reduces the likelihood of human error and allows physicians to come up with a precise treatment plan. The algorithms of AI also have the ability to accurately identify a wide variety of pathologies such as valvopathies and ischemia with coronary artery disease. In fact, Zhang et al. was able to use AI to accurately identify 96% of parasternal long axis imaging views from echocardiography [22]. The use of AI to improve the diagnostic ability of echocardiograms is still in its early stages and research is still in progress before it becomes more widespread [23].

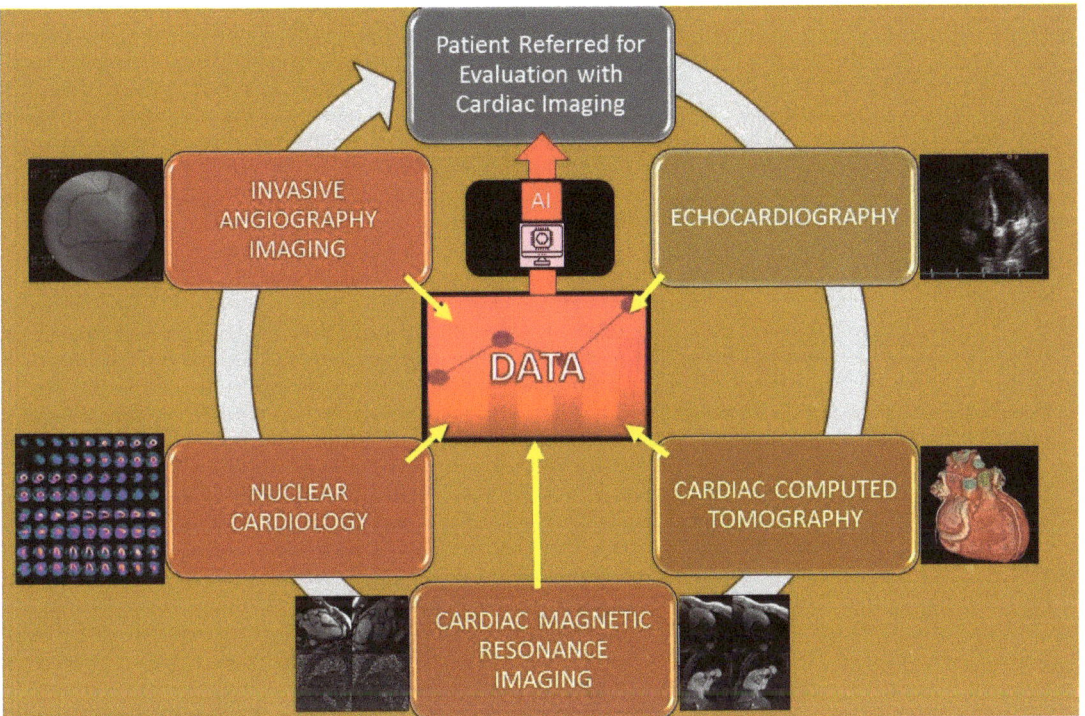

Figure 2. Cardiac imaging modalities that allow for the gathering of data that informs the formation of artificial intelligence that then is used for optimization of the evaluation of patients undergoing cardiac imaging.

It is often difficult to distinguish between several conditions on echocardiography. Narula et al. states how machine learning can be applied to echocardiography to help differentiate between hypertrophic cardiomyopathy and athlete's heart [24]. Machine learning algorithms are also particularly beneficial to help streamline workflow and prevent errors from physicians reading images after experiencing fatigue and exhaustion. Specifically, Madani et al. applied a CNN algorithm model to 267 echocardiogram images with 15 standard views and trained the algorithm by using labeled images. The results found that the model was immediately able to identify the echocardiogram view with an accuracy of 97.8% as compared to 70.2–84% accuracy with readings by expert echocardiographers [25].

3.2. Cardiac Computed Tomography

In addition to echocardiography, computed tomography (CT) is also a valuable imaging tool for cardiovascular diseases. The CT scan produces images of the heart in various planes and allows for 3D image generation. It is particularly applicable for patients with suspected CAD as CT imaging allows physicians to noninvasively assess for calcium and plaque presence in the coronary arteries. This would indicate the presence of a blockage or narrowing in the arteries due to plaque buildup [26]. The amount of calcium in the vessels, also referred to as calcium score, can indicate the extent and prognosis of CAD. A study by Al'Aref et al. used machine learning algorithms to combine the calcium score and clinical factors to predict CAD in 35,281 patients. It was found that machine learning in conjunction with the coronary artery calcium score resulted in the most significantly accurate assessment of obstructive CAD from CT imaging compared to machine learning or calcium score alone [27]. Machine learning has been used to identify a variety of different pathologies on CT with accuracy [28].

Furthermore, machine learning allows for low-dose CT scans to be safer. Low-dose CT imaging brings concerns of increased exposure to radiation for patients that could not be solved by simply decreasing radiation levels as this would decrease the image quality [29]. As a result, to solve this issue, a machine learning framework was developed that allowed for reconstructing image parameters and denoising the quality of the image when low radiation was used. This resulted in improved image quality to equate to the regular-dose CT image quality, thus allowing patients to be exposed to less radiation while still obtaining a diagnostic result [30].

3.3. Cardiac Magnetic Resonance Imaging

Cardiac magnetic resonance imaging (MRI) is another noninvasive diagnostic tool for assessing cardiovascular diseases. Specifically, the MRI is considered the gold standard for assessing the ejection fraction and left ventricular volume [31]. In a study by Ruijsink et al., researchers found a high correlation between the deep learning algorithm and manual analysis of the left and right ventricular volumes, filling, and ejection rates [31]. In turn, automated measurements through deep learning were seen to be in strong agreement with the manual interpretation. Particularly, deep learning can be used to reconstruct cardiac images with better 3D visualization to identify disease patterns in association with the right ventricle. This is because the right ventricle is often not easily visualized in 2D with echocardiography. Laser et al. found that reconstruction of the right ventricle with echocardiography and cardiac MRI had incredible accuracy and reproducibility compared to the gold standard direct cardiac MRI [32]. Deep learning also allows for the extraction of specific features to be automated easily, such as identification of the right ventricle and pulmonary artery hypertension [19,33,34]. A study by Zhang et al. created a deep learning model that created the ability to obtain motion features from the left ventricle and discriminate between ischemic regions on a nonenhanced cardiac MRI. This deep learning framework is beneficial as it allows for confirmation of chronic myocardial infarctions on MRI [35].

Cardiac MRI has increasingly been used as a noninvasive imaging tool over the years. It results in acquiring cross-sectional images aligned with the heart axes. This can pose as an additional challenge when reading MRI results as medical imaging experts require detailed knowledge on cardiac anatomy. Conventionally, the heart is automatically localized to the center of the image, which does not account for the diversity in various patients' anatomy. This assumption leads to lower sensitivity and potential errors in imaging results [9]. Kabani et al. introduced CNN, or deep neural network application, which allows for localizing and detecting a region of interest on an MRI interest. Normally, most localization networks have a bounding box around the region of interest. In this case, the CNN neural network applied a classification task where each pixel in the image was a separate class. Then, the CNN was trained to determine where the object was in the image and classify the pixels as in the background or in the bounding box. Specifically, this neural network considered the problem as a classification task where the pixels were classified as in the background or in a box [8].

3.4. Nuclear Cardiology

Nuclear cardiology uses noninvasive techniques to measure blood flow through the heart. This test is particularly applicable when diagnosing coronary artery disease and possible ischemia, or lack of oxygen to the heart due to decreased blood flow. There are two types of nuclear cardiology tests that can be performed, the cardiac SPECT and PET-CT.

In both tests, a PET scan is formed following injection of radioactive chemicals into the bloodstream via IV [36]. Artificial intelligence, particularly deep learning, can also be applied to nuclear cardiology in order to address disparities regarding the diagnostic ability of SPECT [19]. Deep learning allows for a greater ability to analyze images by identifying high dimensional patterns. Juarez-Orozco et al. applied deep learning to evaluate perfusion polar maps in ischemia by PET. It was found that deep learning had an area under the receiver-operating curve (AUC) of 0.90, which was better than all comparator models [19]. Additionally, Hu et al. implemented the subset of AI, machine learning, to predict the likelihood of early coronary revascularization within 90 days after SPECT imaging. When comparing the AUC of machine learning with the standard quantitative analysis, it was found that the AUC of early coronary revascularization prediction was higher than and outperformed that of standard quantitative analysis [37].

3.5. Angiography Imaging

Another imaging tool used in the field of cardiology is invasive angiography imaging. This is considered the reference standard when diagnosing obstructive coronary artery disease as it provides a detailed outlook on the structure and function of the heart's blood vessels. Despite its benefits, there are risks associated with the invasive angiography procedure including serious complications as well as expensive costs, exposure to high radiation, and discomfort [38]. As such, Wolterink et al. validated a feasible method to obtain reduced radiation dose CT images by training a deep learning model [39]. This shows how deep learning can help improve diagnostic imaging tools as well to make procedures safer for patients while also providing more accurate results.

Furthermore, cardiac computed tomography angiography (CCTA) is another method to diagnose coronary artery disease. Although CCTA can be used to rule out CAD, there are many drawbacks to using this diagnostic tool as it overestimates the amount of stenosis of the vessel and takes a lot of time to yield results. However, with the addition of AI, CCTA can be significantly improved to result in a more accurate evaluation of coronary stenosis, plaque characterization, and degree of myocardial ischemia [40]. For example, van Hamersvelt et al. evaluated the addition of deep learning algorithm to analyze the left ventricular myocardium in CCTA for degree of stenosis. It was found that there was improved diagnosis and identification of patients with functionally significant coronary artery stenosis when using CCTA in combination with deep learning analysis. Specifically, sensitivity and specificity of results were 84.6% and 48.4%, respectively [41].

Motwani et al. applied machine learning to evaluate 5-year all-cause mortality in patients undergoing CCTA [42]. Specifically, 10,030 patients with possible CAD underwent CCTA as part of their standard of care. Machine learning was then applied to predict 5-year mortality of these patients using the CCTA data. After comparison of a 5-year follow-up from these patients via the CCTA international multicenter registry, it was found that ML combined with CCTA data was significantly better at predicting patient prognosis for the next 5 years compared to CCTA metrics alone [42].

ML-based fractional flow reserve-computed tomography (FFR-CT) is increasingly used in diagnosing CAD. Specifically, FFR-CT is a noninvasive procedure that generates a 3D image of the patient's coronary arteries [43]. An FFR measurement refers to identifying the ratio between the maximum blood flow possible in a diseased coronary artery and maximum flow in a normal coronary artery. An FFR of 1.0 is considered normal whereas an FFR of less than 0.75–0.80 is associated with myocardial ischemia [44]. A study by Jiang et al. evaluated the features and severity of coronary calcification by ML-based CCTA-derived FFR, or FFR-CT. In this study, 442 patients went through CCTA, ML-based FFR-CT, and invasive FFR and the results were compared. It was found that ML-based FFR-CT had an accuracy of 0.90 in determining calcification lesions as compared to invasive FFR. Additionally, CT-FFR generally had higher accuracy in diagnosis and differentiating ischemia in blood vessels as compared to CCTA by itself [45].

A study by Yang et al. analyzed the relation of stenosis and plaque characteristics with myocardial implications. The study analyzed 1013 vessels via fractional flow reserve measurement and CT angiography. Then, Yang et al. incorporated machine learning to identify the features associated with a low FFR and the patient prognosis. In this case, machine learning was beneficial in categorizing characteristics of blood vessels with a low FFR. The six functionally relevant features found included minimum lumen area, percent atheroma volume, fibrofatty and necrotic core volume, plaque volume, proximal left anterior descending coronary artery lesion, and remodeling index [46].

3.6. Intravascular Imaging

Intravascular imaging is performed by using a specialized catheter-based intravascular ultrasound (IVUS) or optical coherence tomography (OCT) that allows for providing a real-time visual of the inside of a coronary artery. Particularly, it shows the degree of narrowing or thickening of an artery and a visual of the lumen of the artery. Intravascular ultrasound is often used to gain a better insight into the nature of the plaque in the artery as well as in the placement of stents [47]. This imaging technique is invasive and involves great expertise to place the catheters inside the coronary arteries. Researchers have incorporated artificial intelligence to increase the speed of diagnosis and interpretation of intravascular imaging in real time [48]. Specifically, the artificial intelligence algorithm is exposed to multiple images and given information on each image, such as the vessel's geometry and distribution of different tissue types. Therefore, as it is exposed to more images, the AI algorithm can easily and quickly interpret the image created by the intravascular imaging and discern a diagnosis.

IVUS imaging creates an image with low resolution but with high tissue penetration while OCT imaging creates an image with higher resolution but limited tissue penetration. As these two intravascular imaging modalities have their differences, artificial intelligence can connect the two results together. Specifically, AI processes data from IVUS and OCT images into a single imaging procedure to allow physicians to review all the data at once [48]. This is beneficial as it allows for a more rapid, comprehensive evaluation of any damaged arteries.

3.7. Software Programs in Clinical Practice That Employ AI

Artificial intelligence is already being used in clinical practice by physicians today. There are software programs, such as IBM Watson®, that help organizations automate complex processes to improve efficiency and effectivity. IBM Watson® includes Merge Healthcare®, which provides medical imaging artificial intelligence solutions to help physicians with patient care. Specifically, Merge PACS™ is an artificial-intelligence-ready workflow platform that eases the physician workload of reading and understanding numerous dense images [49]. This is extremely beneficial as physicians have received an increasing number of images to read over the years, including as many as 100,000 images a day [50]. Therefore, artificial intelligence and computer programming offered through Merge Healthcare® serves to provide a more rapid and automated diagnosis for patients.

4. Limitations of Artificial Intelligence

Overall, AI applications mimic human intelligence with the purpose of solving problems or making decisions. AI has many advantages with its accuracy, cost-effectiveness, and reliability. However, there are still some limitations to AI, especially with its application in the medical field. Specifically, the gold standard for clinical reasoning in decision making should still be at the physicians' discretion. Since AI results in producing automated decisions, this can lead to a decision-making bias as physicians can be more likely to trust diagnostic test results by AI-led machines without intense scrutiny [33]. Consequently, there is a gray area as to with whom the responsibility lies in the case of an error. Data interpretation with AI can be susceptible to selection bias as well [34]. This is because the results AI produces are dependent upon the data entered. Therefore, if there is poor data entry, the results lead to invalid assumptions without a fair, accurate representation. Furthermore, another limitation of newer models of AI is the ability to reproduce and standardize the method [34,51,52]. It is difficult to compare diagnostic results from different providers if they are analyzing the data with varying techniques.

5. Future Applications of Artificial Intelligence

As newer techniques are emerging, AI is constantly expanding beyond its limits and capabilities. Within the field of medicine, it has the potential to lead to newer advances in drug therapies as well as diagnoses of diseases at an earlier stage [34]. It is anticipated that AI will have the ability in the future to fully automate reading echocardiography images and detecting pathology [32]. Furthermore, it allows treatment plans to become more standardized based on an automated process. With AI completing tasks at a quicker rate, physicians have more time to be free from mundane tasks such as data input and electronic health records to focus on educating the patient and fostering a stronger patient–physician relationship [32]. Although AI holds great potential for the future of medicine, physicians should still be responsible for making the final clinical judgment.

6. Conclusions

Artificial intelligence allows for the potential to expand and improve medical technologies for better patient care. Specifically, the ability of the algorithms to make diagnoses more accurate is useful for physicians to detect diseases earlier in their course to plan for the right treatment action. Within AI, the branch of machine learning has been prevalent in the field of cardiology. This is because there are a variety of imaging tools implemented when conducting a patient workup. In the future, AI will continue to expand and become more accurate in giving an ideal diagnosis for improved decision making as technology progresses and the dataset available to form algorithms and identify patterns becomes larger.

Funding: This research received no external funding.

Conflicts of Interest: The authors declare no conflict of interest.

References

1. Itchhaporia, D. Artificial intelligence in cardiology. *Trends Cardiovasc. Med.* **2020**, *32*, 34–41. [CrossRef]
2. Zhang, X.-D. Machine learning. In *A Matrix Algebra Approach to Artificial Intelligence*; Springer: Singapore, 2020; pp. 223–440.
3. Supervised vs. Unsupervised Learning—Javatpoint. Available online: https://www.javatpoint.com/difference-between-supervised-and-unsupervised-learning (accessed on 28 October 2021).
4. IBM Cloud Education. What is Supervised Learning? IBM. Available online: https://www.ibm.com/cloud/learn/supervised-learning (accessed on 23 December 2021).
5. IBM. Supervised vs. Unsupervised Learning: What's the Difference? Available online: https://www.ibm.com/cloud/blog/supervised-vs-unsupervised-learning (accessed on 9 January 2021).
6. Yu, A.C.; Eng, J. One Algorithm May Not Fit All: How Selection Bias Affects Machine Learning Performance. *RadioGraphics* **2020**, *40*, 1932–1937. [CrossRef]
7. Buch, V.H.; Ahmed, I.; Maruthappu, M. Artificial intelligence in medicine: Current trends and future possibilities. *Br. J. Gen. Pr.* **2018**, *68*, 143–144. [CrossRef]
8. Kabani, A.; El-Sakka, M.R. Object Detection and Localization Using Deep Convolutional Networks with Softmax Activation and Multi-class Log Loss. In *Image Analysis and Recognition*; Campilho, A., Karray, F., Eds.; Springer International Publishing: Cham, Switzerland, 2016; pp. 358–366.
9. Arafati, A.; Hu, P.; Finn, J.P.; Rickers, C.; Cheng, A.L.; Jafarkhani, H.; Kheradvar, A. Artificial intelligence in pediatric and adult congenital cardiac MRI: An unmet clinical need. *Cardiovasc. Diagn. Ther.* **2019**, *9*, S310–S325. [CrossRef]
10. Shah, S.J.; Katz, D.; Selvaraj, S.; Burke, M.A.; Yancy, C.W.; Gheorghiade, M.; Bonow, R.O.; Huang, C.-C.; Deo, R.C. Phenomapping for Novel Classification of Heart Failure with Preserved Ejection Fraction. *Circulation* **2015**, *131*, 269–279. [CrossRef]
11. West, D.M. What is Artificial Intelligence? Brookings Institution. 2019. Available online: https://www.brookings.edu/research/what-is-artificial-intelligence/ (accessed on 28 October 2021).
12. Lim, L.J.; Tison, G.H.; Delling, F.N. Artificial Intelligence in Cardiovascular Imaging. *Methodist DeBakey Cardiovasc. J.* **2020**, *16*, 138–145. [CrossRef]
13. Hamet, P.; Tremblay, J. Artificial Intelligence in medicine. *Metabolism* **2017**, *69*, S36–S40. [CrossRef]

14. Amisha, P.M.; Pathania, M.; Rathaur, V.K. Overview of artificial intelligence in medicine. *J. Fam. Med. Prim. Care* **2019**, *8*, 2328–2331. [CrossRef]
15. Momentum Janitorial. Ai-Enabled Robotic Surgery: How Collaborative Robots are Assisting Surgeons. Far North Surgery. 18 October 2020. Available online: https://www.farnorthsurgery.com/blog/aienabled-robotic-surgery-how-collaborative-robots-are-assisting-surgeons (accessed on 23 December 2021).
16. Study Identifies Human Errors Associated with Surgical Errors. Baylor College of Medicine. Available online: https://www.bcm.edu/news/human-errors-adverse-surgical-events (accessed on 28 October 2021).
17. Gottdiener, J.S.; Bednarz, J.; Devereux, R.; Gardin, J.; Klein, A.; Manning, W.J.; Morehead, A.; Kitzman, D.; Oh, J.; Quinones, M.; et al. American Society of Echocardiography recommendations for use of echocardiography in clinical trials. *J. Am. Soc. Echocardiogr.* **2004**, *17*, 1086–1119. [CrossRef]
18. Rajih, E.; Tholomier, C.; Cormier, B.; Samouëlian, V.; Warkus, T.; Liberman, M.; Widmer, H.; Lattouf, J.-B.; Alenizi, A.M.; Meskawi, M.; et al. Error reporting from the da Vinci surgical system in robotic surgery: A Canadian multispecialty experience at a single academic centre. *Can. Urol. Assoc. J.* **2017**, *11*, E197–E202. [CrossRef]
19. Seetharam, K.; Brito, D.; Farjo, P.D.; Sengupta, P.P. The Role of Artificial Intelligence in Cardiovascular Imaging: State of the Art Review. *Front. Cardiovasc. Med.* **2020**, *7*, 618849. [CrossRef]
20. Arsanjani, R.; Xu, Y.; Dey, D.; Fish, M.; Dorbala, S.; Hayes, S.; Berman, D.; Germano, G.; Slomka, P. Improved Accuracy of Myocardial Perfusion SPECT for the Detection of Coronary Artery Disease Using a Support Vector Machine Algorithm. *J. Nucl. Med.* **2013**, *54*, 549–555. [CrossRef]
21. Seetharam, K.; Shrestha, S.; Mills, J.D.; Sengupta, P.P. Artificial Intelligence in Nuclear Cardiology: Adding Value to Prognostication. *Curr. Cardiovasc. Imaging Rep.* **2019**, *12*, 14. [CrossRef]
22. Zhang, J.; Gajjala, S.; Agrawal, P.; Tison, G.H.; Hallock, L.A.; Beussink-Nelson, L.; Lassen, M.H.; Fan, E.; Aras, M.A.; Jordan, C.; et al. Fully Automated Echocardiogram Interpretation in Clinical Practice. *Circulation* **2018**, *138*, 1623–1635. [CrossRef]
23. Alsharqi, M.; Woodward, W.; Mumith, A.; Markham, D.; Upton, R.; Leeson, P. Artificial intelligence and echocardiography. *Echo Res. Pract.* **2018**, *5*, R115–R125. [CrossRef]
24. Narula, S.; Shameer, K.; Omar, A.M.S.; Dudley, J.T.; Sengupta, P.P. Machine-Learning Algorithms to Automate Morphological and Functional Assessments in 2D Echocardiography. *J. Am. Coll. Cardiol.* **2016**, *68*, 2287–2295. [CrossRef]
25. Seetharam, K.; Raina, S.; Sengupta, P.P. The Role of Artificial Intelligence in Echocardiography. *Curr. Cardiol. Rep.* **2020**, *22*, 99. [CrossRef] [PubMed]
26. ACR RSNA. Cardiac CT for Calcium Scoring. Radiologyinfo.org 2020. Available online: https://www.radiologyinfo.org/en/info/ct_calscoring (accessed on 28 October 2021).
27. Al'Aref, S.J.; Maliakal, G.; Singh, G.; van Rosendael, A.R.; Ma, X.; Xu, Z.; Alawamlh, O.A.H.; Lee, B.; Pandey, M.; Achenbach, S.; et al. Machine learning of clinical variables and coronary artery calcium scoring for the prediction of obstructive coronary artery disease on coronary computed tomography angiography: Analysis from the CONFIRM registry. *Eur. Heart J.* **2019**, *41*, 359–367. [CrossRef] [PubMed]
28. Lin, A.; Kolossváry, M.; Motwani, M.; Išgum, I.; Maurovich-Horvat, P.; Slomka, P.J.; Dey, D. Artificial intelligence in cardiovascular CT: Current status and future implications. *J. Cardiovasc. Comput. Tomogr.* **2021**, *15*, 462–469. [CrossRef]
29. McCollough, C.; Leng, S. Use of artificial intelligence in computed tomography dose optimisation. *Ann. ICRP* **2020**, *49*, 113–125. [CrossRef]
30. Immonen, E.; Wong, J.; Nieminen, M.; Kekkonen, L.; Roine, S.; Törnroos, S.; Lanca, L.; Guan, F.; Metsälä, E. The use of deep learning towards dose optimization in low-dose computed tomography: A scoping review. *Radiography* **2021**, *28*, 208–214. [CrossRef] [PubMed]
31. Seetharam, K.; Kagiyama, N.; Shrestha, S.; Sengupta, P.P. Clinical Inference From Cardiovascular Imaging: Paradigm Shift Towards Machine-Based Intelligent Platform. *Curr. Treat. Options Cardiovasc. Med.* **2020**, *22*, 8. [CrossRef]
32. Kuehn, B.M. Cardiac Imaging on the Cusp of an Artificial Intelligence Revolution. *Circulation* **2020**, *141*, 1266–1267. [CrossRef] [PubMed]
33. Dorado-Díaz, P.I.; Sampedro-Gómez, J.; Vicente-Palacios, V.; Sánchez, P.L. Applications of Artificial Intelligence in Cardiology. The Future is Already Here. *Rev. Española Cardiol.* **2019**, *72*, 1065–1075. [CrossRef]
34. Mathur, P.; Srivastava, S.; Xu, X.; Mehta, J.L. Artificial Intelligence, Machine Learning, and Cardiovascular Disease. *Clin. Med. Insights Cardiol.* **2020**, *14*. [CrossRef]
35. Zhang, N.; Yang, G.; Gao, Z.; Xu, C.; Zhang, Y.; Shi, R.; Keegan, J.; Xu, L.; Zhang, H.; Fan, Z.; et al. Deep learning for diagnosis of chronic myocardial infarction on nonen-hanced cardiac cine MRI. *Radiology* **2019**, *291*, 606–617. [CrossRef]
36. El-Tallawi, K.C.; Aljizeeri, A.; Nabi, F.; Al-Mallah, M.H. Myocardial Perfusion Imaging Using Positron Emission Tomography. *Methodist DeBakey Cardiovasc. J.* **2020**, *16*, 114–121. [CrossRef] [PubMed]
37. Hu, L.-H.; Betancur, J.; Sharir, T.; Einstein, A.J.; Bokhari, S.; Fish, M.B.; Ruddy, T.D.; Kaufmann, P.A.; Sinusas, A.J.; Miller, E.; et al. Machine learning predicts per-vessel early coronary revascularization after fast myocardial perfusion SPECT: Results from multicentre REFINE SPECT registry. *Eur. Heart J. Cardiovasc. Imaging* **2019**, *21*, 549–559. [CrossRef]
38. Knaapen, P. Computed Tomography to Replace Invasive Coronary Angiography? *Circ. Cardiovasc. Imaging* **2019**, *12*, e008710. [CrossRef]

39. Siegersma, K.; Leiner, T.; Chew, D.; Appelman, Y.; Hofstra, L.; Verjans, J. Artificial intelligence in cardiovascular imaging: State of the art and implications for the imaging cardiologist. *Neth. Heart J.* **2019**, *27*, 403–413. [CrossRef]
40. Muscogiuri, G.; Van Assen, M.; Tesche, C.; De Cecco, C.N.; Chiesa, M.; Scafuri, S.; Guglielmo, M.; Baggiano, A.; Fusini, L.; Guaricci, A.I.; et al. Artificial Intelligence in Coronary Computed Tomography Angiography: From Anatomy to Prognosis. *BioMed Res. Int.* **2020**, *2020*, 6649410. [CrossRef]
41. Van Hamersvelt, R.W.; Zreik, M.; Voskuil, M.; Viergever, M.A.; Išgum, I.; Leiner, T. Deep learning analysis of left ventricular myocardium in CT angiographic intermediate-degree coronary stenosis improves the diagnostic accuracy for identification of functionally significant stenosis. *Eur. Radiol.* **2018**, *29*, 2350–2359. [CrossRef] [PubMed]
42. Motwani, M.; Dey, D.; Berman, D.S.; Germano, G.; Achenbach, S.; Al-Mallah, M.; Andreini, D.; Budoff, M.J.; Cademartiri, F.; Callister, T.Q.; et al. Machine learning for prediction of all-cause mortality in patients with suspected coronary artery disease: A 5-year multicentre prospective registry analysis. *Eur. Heart J.* **2016**, *38*, 500–507. [CrossRef] [PubMed]
43. Fractional Flow Reserve—Computed Tomography: Heart Care in NJ. RWJBarnabas Health. Available online: https://www.rwjbh.org/treatment-care/heart-and-vascular-care/tests-procedures/fractional-flow-reserve-computed-tomography/ (accessed on 9 January 2022).
44. Eiman Jahangir, M.D.; Fractional Flow Reserve (FFR) Measurement. Fractional Flow Reserve (FFR) Measurement. Background, Indications, Outcomes. Background, Indications, Outcomes. Medscape, 2021. Available online: https://emedicine.medscape.com/article/1839601-overview#a1 (accessed on 9 January 2022).
45. Di Jiang, M.; Zhang, X.L.; Liu, H.; Tang, C.X.; Li, J.H.; Wang, Y.N.; Xu, P.P.; Zhou, C.S.; Zhou, F.; Lu, M.J.; et al. The effect of coronary calcification on diagnostic performance of machine learning–based CT-FFR: A Chinese multicenter study. *Eur. Radiol.* **2020**, *31*, 1482–1493. [CrossRef]
46. Yang, S.; Koo, B.-K.; Hoshino, M.; Lee, J.M.; Murai, T.; Park, J.; Zhang, J.; Hwang, D.; Shin, E.-S.; Doh, J.-H.; et al. CT Angiographic and Plaque Predictors of Functionally Significant Coronary Disease and Outcome Using Machine Learning. *JACC Cardiovasc. Imaging* **2020**, *14*, 629–641. [CrossRef] [PubMed]
47. Intravascular Ultrasound (IVUS). Cedars. Available online: https://www.cedars-sinai.org/programs/heart/clinical/womens-heart/services/ivus-intravascular-ultrasound.html (accessed on 9 January 2022).
48. Using AI to Facilitate Diagnosis. Harvard-MIT Health Sciences and Technology. 2021. Available online: https://hst.mit.edu/news-events/using-ai-facilitate-diagnosis (accessed on 9 January 2022).
49. Merge PACS—Overview. IBM. (n.d.). Available online: https://www.ibm.com/products/merge-pacs (accessed on 14 November 2021).
50. Miller, R. IBM Buying Merge Healthcare for $1B to Bring Medical Image Analysis to Watson Health. TechCrunch. 6 August 2015. Available online: https://techcrunch.com/2015/08/06/ibm-buying-merge-healthcare-for-1b to bring-medical-image-analysis-to-watson-health/ (accessed on 14 November 2021).
51. Shameer, K.; Johnson, K.; Glicksberg, B.; Dudley, J.T.; Sengupta, P.P. Machine learning in cardiovascular medicine: Are we there yet? *Heart* **2018**, *104*, 1156–1164. [CrossRef] [PubMed]
52. Al'Aref, S.J.; Anchouche, K.; Singh, G.; Slomka, P.J.; Kolli, K.K.; Kumar, A.; Pandey, M.; Maliakal, G.; van Rosendael, A.R.; Beecy, A.N.; et al. Clinical applications of machine learning in cardiovascular disease and its relevance to cardiac imaging. *Eur. Heart J.* **2019**, *40*, 1975–1986. [CrossRef]

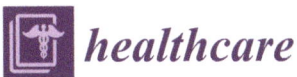

Comment

Comment on Patel, B.; Makaryus, A.N. Artificial Intelligence Advances in the World of Cardiovascular Imaging. *Healthcare* 2022, *10*, 154

Daniele Giansanti

Centro Nazionale Tecnologie Innovative in Sanità Pubblica, Istituto Superiore di Sanità, 00161 Rome, Italy; daniele.giansanti@iss.it; Tel.: +39-06-49902701

Citation: Giansanti, D. Comment on Patel, B.; Makaryus, A.N. Artificial Intelligence Advances in the World of Cardiovascular Imaging. *Healthcare* 2022, *10*, 154. *Healthcare* **2022**, *10*, 727. https://doi.org/10.3390/healthcare10040727

Academic Editor: Norbert Hosten

Received: 23 January 2022
Accepted: 7 April 2022
Published: 14 April 2022

Publisher's Note: MDPI stays neutral with regard to jurisdictional claims in published maps and institutional affiliations.

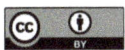

Copyright: © 2022 by the author. Licensee MDPI, Basel, Switzerland. This article is an open access article distributed under the terms and conditions of the Creative Commons Attribution (CC BY) license (https://creativecommons.org/licenses/by/4.0/).

Regarding Dr. Makaryus's interesting review study [1], I would like to express my opinion on it.

I found that this work is particularly stimulating and that it gives a great deal of added value to the Special Issue *"The Artificial Intelligence in Digital Pathology and Digital Radiology: Where Are We?"* [2,3].

Specifically, I believe that this review has the great merit of focusing on the developments of Artificial Intelligence (AI) in the field of *Digital Cardiology* (DC), in a medical sector as broad and strategic as that of cardiology. Many of the considerations that emerge from the review in this specific sector of *Digital Radiology* (DR), such as those relating to the imaging, are exportable to the entire sector. From the review [1], it emerges clearly that the introduction of artificial intelligence (AI) into the world of digital cardiovascular imaging is greatly broadening the capabilities of the field, both with respect to advancements as well as with respect to the complete and accurate diagnosis of cardiovascular conditions. Among the application sectors in which the review [2] has shown the greatest potential we find recognition, diagnostics, protocol automation, and quality control for the analysis of cardiovascular imaging modalities such as, cardiovascular computed tomography, cardiovascular magnetic resonance imaging, nuclear cardiac imaging, echocardiography, and other sectors of imaging. All this is in line with what emerges in the field of DR [4] in general. All this will lead to important changes in the organization of work and to continuous challenges that will involve all actors, such as the radiologist, the hemodynamist, the cardiologist, the general practitioner, the medical radiology technician, and other professionals and patients. In DR [4], AI will be useful for: simplifying all the management activities, from the scheduling of the patients up to the reports and the bill; medical decision support in a specific imaging application; suggesting the most appropriate exam after a scrutiny of the patient's virtual directory; both cleaning/de-noising the signal and minimizing the artifact; facilitating the automated image interpretation; and dimensional and volumetric measurements.

To support the insiders in medical activity, data science specialists work on the development of increasingly better performing and targeted algorithms that must be calibrated considering the specificity of the application, the decision-making protocols and the physical process which is different in the formation of images. For this reason, it is important that the insiders talk with these scientific scholars who are also involved in basic research both to give new stimuli and to give feedback on use.

Precisely because of the challenges and changes taking place, in [5] it was highlighted that some studies are addressing in a targeted manner aspects relating to the acceptance and consent of the introduction of AI in DR. These studies, also reported in [5], are mainly based on questionnaires carried out in an original way, and only in rare cases are these questionnaires of a standardized type [6–20].

Among the various potentials that this type of investigation has, in addition to providing important outputs on the integration agreement of AI in DR, we find those of raising awareness among stakeholders and putting data science specialists in communication with insiders.

These studies reported in [5] concerned all the professionals involved. The results highlighted, among other things: the importance of both looking at these professionals in a comparative and single way; to deal in a broad and detailed way with the applications of DR impacted by AI; and the need to be supported by scientific societies and by federations of scientific societies.

I tried to see if such activities have started in the DC sector, by means of a preliminary and rapid search.

I made the following two queries on the Pubmed database:

- Search: ((Artificial Intelligence[Title/Abstract]) AND (Cardiology[Title/Abstract])) AND (consensus [Title/Abstract]) [21].
- Search: ((Artificial Intelligence[Title/Abstract]) AND (Cardiology[Title/Abstract])) AND (acceptance[Title/Abstract]) [22].

I found four studies; however, they did not address the issue of *acceptance* and *consensus* specifically.

I would like to ask you if you believe that, among the future work in the integration activities of AI in cardiology in the applications and sectors that you highlighted very clearly in the review, there will be a need for desirable and/or possible acceptance and consensus initiatives based on targeted investigations on insiders and, if so, if you believe that also in this case, by analogy to the DR in general, they will be based on survey tools, such as the questionnaires used in DR and with a similar approach [5].

Funding: This research received no external funding.

Institutional Review Board Statement: Not applicable.

Informed Consent Statement: Not applicable.

Data Availability Statement: Not applicable.

Conflicts of Interest: The authors declare no conflict of interest.

References

1. Patel, B.; Makaryus, A.N. Artificial Intelligence Advances in the World of Cardiovascular Imaging. *Healthcare* **2022**, *10*, 154. [CrossRef] [PubMed]
2. Available online: https://www.mdpi.com/journal/healthcare/special_issues/AI_Digital_Pathology_Radiology (accessed on 6 April 2022).
3. Giansanti, D. The Artificial Intelligence in Digital Pathology and Digital Radiology: Where Are We? *Healthcare* **2021**, *9*, 30. [CrossRef] [PubMed]
4. Gampala, S.; Vankeshwaram, V.; Gadula, S.S.P. Is Artificial Intelligence the New Friend for Radiologists? A Review Article. *Cureus* **2020**, *12*, e11137. [CrossRef] [PubMed]
5. Di Basilio, F.; Esposito, G.; Monoscalco, L.; Giansanti, D. The Artificial Intelligence in Digital Radiology: Part 2: Towards an Investigation of acceptance and consensus on the Insiders. *Healthcare* **2022**, *10*, 153. [CrossRef] [PubMed]
6. Lennartz, S.; Dratsch, T.; Zopfs, D.; Persigehl, T.; Maintz, D.; Hokamp, N.G.; dos Santos, D.P. Use and Control of Artificial Intelligence in Patients across the Medical Workflow: Single-Center Questionnaire Study of Patient Perspectives. *J. Med. Internet Res.* **2021**, *23*, e24221. [CrossRef] [PubMed]
7. Zhang, Z.; Citardi, D.; Wang, D.; Genc, Y.; Shan, J.; Fan, X. Patients' perceptions of using artificial intelligence (AI)-based technology to comprehend radiology imaging data. *Health Inform. J.* **2021**, *27*, 14604582211011215. [CrossRef] [PubMed]
8. Ongena, Y.P.; Haan, M.; Yakar, D.; Kwee, T.C. Patients' views on the implementation of artificial intelligence in radiology: Development and validation of a standardized questionnaire. *Eur. Radiol.* **2020**, *30*, 1033–1040. [CrossRef] [PubMed]
9. Hendrix, N.; Hauber, B.; Lee, C.I.; Bansal, A.; Veenstra, D.L. Artificial intelligence in breast cancer screening: Primary care provider preferences. *J. Am. Med. Inform. Assoc.* **2021**, *28*, 1117–1124. [CrossRef] [PubMed]
10. Abuzaid, M.M.; Elshami, W.; McConnell, J.; Tekin, H.O. An extensive survey oradiographers from the Middle East and India on artificial intelligence integration in radiology practice. *Health Technol.* **2021**, *11*, 1045–1050. [CrossRef] [PubMed]
11. Abuzaid, M.M.; Tekin, H.O.; Reza, M.; Elhag, I.R.; Elshami, W. Assessment of MRI technologists in acceptance and willingness to integrate artificial intelligence into practice. *Radiography* **2021**, *27*, S83–S87. [CrossRef] [PubMed]

12. Giansanti, D.; Rossi., I.; Monoscalco, L. Lessons from the COVID-19 Pandemic on the Use of Artificial Intelligence in Digital Radiology: The Submission of a Survey to Investigate the Opinion of Insiders. *Healthcare* **2021**, *9*, 331. [CrossRef] [PubMed]
13. Abuzaid, M.M.; Elshami, W.; Tekin, H.; Issa, B. Assessment of the Willingness of Radiologists and Radiographers to Accept the Integration of Artificial Intelligence into Radiology Practice. *Acad. Radiol.* **2020**, *29*, 87–94. [CrossRef] [PubMed]
14. Alelyani, M.; Alamri, S.; Alqahtani, M.S.; Musa, A.; Almater, H.; Alqahtani, N.; Alshahrani, F.; Alelyani, S. Radiology Community Attitude in Saudi Arabia about the Applications of Artificial Intelligence in Radiology. *Healthcare* **2021**, *9*, 834. [CrossRef] [PubMed]
15. European Society of Radiology (ESR). Impact of artificial intelligence on radiology: A EuroAIM survey among members of the European Society of Radiology. *Insights Imaging* **2019**, *10*, 105. [CrossRef] [PubMed]
16. Galán, C.; Portero, F.S. Medical students' perceptions of the impact of artificial intelligence in Radiology. *Radiologia* **2021**. [CrossRef]
17. Aldosari, B. User acceptance of a picture archiving and communication system (PACS) in a Saudi Arabian hospital radiology department. *BMC Med. Inform. Decis. Mak.* **2012**, *12*, 44. [CrossRef] [PubMed]
18. Diaz, O.; Guidi, G.; Ivashchenko, O.; Colgan, N.; Zanca, F. Artificial intelligence in the medical physics community: An international survey. *Phys. Med.* **2021**, *81*, 141–146. [CrossRef] [PubMed]
19. Coppola, F.; Faggioni, L.; Regge, D.; Giovagnoni, A.; Golfieri, R.; Bibbolino, C.; Miele, V.; Neri, E.; Grassi, R. Artificial intelli-gence: Radiologists' expectations and opinions gleaned from a nationwide online survey. *Radiol. Med.* **2021**, *126*, 63–71. [CrossRef] [PubMed]
20. Avanzo, M.; Trianni, A.; Botta, F.; Talamonti, C.; Stasi, M.; Iori, M. Artificial Intelligence and the Medical Physicist: Welcome to the Machine. *Appl. Sci.* **2021**, *11*, 1691. [CrossRef]
21. Pubmed Search with Query ": ((Artificial Intelligence[Title/Abstract]) AND (Cardiology[Title/Abstract])) AND (Consensus [Title/Abstract]). Available online: https://pubmed.ncbi.nlm.nih.gov/?term=%28%28Artificial+Intelligence%5BTitle%2FAbstract%5D%29+AND+%28Cardiology%5BTitle%2FAbstract%5D%29%29+AND+%28consensus+%5BTitle%2FAbstract%5D%29&sort=date&size=200 (accessed on 23 January 2022).
22. You Can Add Pubmed Search with Query ": ((Artificial Intelligence[Title/Abstract]) AND (Cardiology[Title/Abstract])) AND (Acceptance[Title/Abstract])". Available online: https://pubmed.ncbi.nlm.nih.gov/?term=%28%28Artificial+Intelligence%5BTitle%2FAbstract%5D%29+AND+%28Cardiology%5BTitle%2FAbstract%5D%29%29+AND+%28acceptance%5BTitle%2FAbstract%5D%29&sort=date&size=200 (accessed on 23 January 2022).

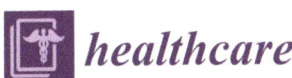

Reply

Reply to Giansanti, D. Comment on "Patel, B.; Makaryus, A.N. Artificial Intelligence Advances in the World of Cardiovascular Imaging. *Healthcare* 2022, 10, 154"

Bhakti Patel [1] and Amgad N. Makaryus [1,2,3,*]

1. Donald and Barbara Zucker School of Medicine at Hofstra/Northwell, Hofstra University, Hempstead, NY 11549, USA; bpatel10@pride.hofstra.edu
2. Department of Cardiology, Nassau University Medical Center, East Meadow, NY 11554, USA
3. Department of Cardiology, Northwell Health, Manhasset, NY 11030, USA
* Correspondence: amakaryus@numc.edu; Tel.: +1-516-296-2567

Thank you for your interest and comment [1] on our "Artificial Intelligence Advances in the World of Cardiovascular Imaging" publication in *Healthcare* [2] in your Special Issue on artificial intelligence (AI) in Digital Pathology and Digital Radiology (DR) [3]. Our paper focused on documenting information regarding the applications and use of AI in cardiovascular imaging modalities. In reference to your comment, we believe that among the future work in the integration activities of AI in cardiology, there will be acceptance and consensus initiatives based on target investigations and evaluations from users of the technology and beneficiaries (patients) of the technology's application. Additionally, similar to what has been seen in digital radiology, these initiatives will likely be conducted through questionnaires [4]. Questionnaires seem to be the standard for gathering information regarding patients' experience and thoughts on the application of artificial intelligence in medicine. A study by Lennartz et al., conducted research where surveys were given ascertaining whether patients preferred a physician or AI's role in performing a clinical task. The results showed that patients preferred physicians in most clinical tasks or a physician overseeing AI applications [5]. In another study by Ongena et al., the patient acceptance of artificial intelligence was assessed through questionnaire responses. It was found that, overall, patients were distrustful of AI and preferred personal interaction and connections [6]. This information from these example surveys is useful in terms of AI applications and expansion for the future, and how this information should be integrated into the field. These publications also show the significance of questionnaires on providing feedback for the use of AI applications in imaging modalities. Learning from the patient viewpoint can bring a different perspective to help improve the technology to be implemented for the best impact. In the future, we believe with more implementation and usage of AI, patients will be more exposed to the benefits of AI that help improve imaging modalities, and perspectives may change towards patient preference for more AI integration. For that reason, the questionnaires are a great way to survey for acceptance and consensus and should be given regularly as more AI is introduced into the field of medicine in general and cardiovascular imaging specifically. We look forward to new advances and insights to the further application of AI in the world of cardiovascular imaging.

Funding: This research received no external funding.

Institutional Review Board Statement: Not applicable.

Informed Consent Statement: Not applicable.

Data Availability Statement: Not applicable.

Conflicts of Interest: The authors declare no conflict of interest.

References

1. Giansanti, D. Comment on Patel, B.; Makaryus, A.N. Artificial Intelligence Advances in the World of Cardiovascular Imaging. *Healthcare* 2022, *10*, 154. *Healthcare* **2022**, *10*, 727. [CrossRef]
2. Patel, B.; Makaryus, A.N. Artificial Intelligence Advances in the World of Cardiovascular Imaging. *Healthcare* **2022**, *10*, 154. [CrossRef] [PubMed]
3. Giansanti, D. The Artificial Intelligence in Digital Pathology and Digital Radiology: Where Are We? *Healthcare* **2021**, *9*, 30. [CrossRef] [PubMed]
4. Di Basilio, F.; Esposisto, G.; Monoscalco, L.; Giansanti, D. The Artificial Intelligence in Digital Radiology: Part 2: Towards an Investigation of acceptance and consensus on the Insiders. *Healthcare* **2022**, *10*, 153. [CrossRef] [PubMed]
5. Lennartz, S.; Dratsch, T.; Zopfs, D.; Persigehl, T.; Maintz, D.; Hokamp, N.G.; Dos Santos, D.P. Use and Control of Artificial Intelligence in Patients Across the Medical Workflow: Single-Center Questionnaire Study of Patient Perspectives. *J. Med. Internet Res.* **2021**, *23*, e24221. [CrossRef] [PubMed]
6. Ongena, Y.P.; Haan, M.; Yakar, D.; Kwee, T.C. Patients' views on the implementation of artificial intelligence in radiology: Development and validation of a standardized questionnaire. *Eur. Radiol.* **2020**, *30*, 1033–1040. [CrossRef] [PubMed]

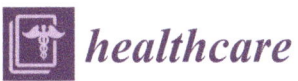

Article

Radiology Community Attitude in Saudi Arabia about the Applications of Artificial Intelligence in Radiology

Magbool Alelyani [1,*], Sultan Alamri [2], Mohammed S. Alqahtani [1], Alamin Musa [1], Hajar Almater [1], Nada Alqahtani [1], Fay Alshahrani [1] and Salem Alelyani [3,4]

1. Department Radiological Sciences, King Khalid University, Abha 61421, Saudi Arabia; mosalqhtani@kku.edu.sa (M.S.A.); aomer@kku.edu.sa (A.M.); 437804506@kku.edu.sa (H.A.); 436803611@kku.edu.sa (N.A.); 437804448@kku.edu.sa (F.A.)
2. Department Radiological Sciences, Taif University, Taif 21944, Saudi Arabia; s.alamri@tu.edu.sa
3. Center for Artificial Intelligence (CAI), King Khalid University, Abha 61421, Saudi Arabia; s.alelyani@kku.edu.sa
4. College of Computer Science, King Khalid University, Abha 61421, Saudi Arabia
* Correspondence: maalalyani@kku.edu.sa

Abstract: Artificial intelligence (AI) is a broad, umbrella term that encompasses the theory and development of computer systems able to perform tasks normally requiring human intelligence. The aim of this study is to assess the radiology community's attitude in Saudi Arabia toward the applications of AI. Methods: Data for this study were collected using electronic questionnaires in 2019 and 2020. The study included a total of 714 participants. Data analysis was performed using SPSS Statistics (version 25). Results: The majority of the participants (61.2%) had read or heard about the role of AI in radiology. We also found that radiologists had statistically different responses and tended to read more about AI compared to all other specialists. In addition, 82% of the participants thought that AI must be included in the curriculum of medical and allied health colleges, and 86% of the participants agreed that AI would be essential in the future. Even though human–machine interaction was considered to be one of the most important skills in the future, 89% of the participants thought that it would never replace radiologists. Conclusion: Because AI plays a vital role in radiology, it is important to ensure that radiologists and radiographers have at least a minimum understanding of the technology. Our finding shows an acceptable level of knowledge regarding AI technology and that AI applications should be included in the curriculum of the medical and health sciences colleges.

Keywords: AI; radiology; awareness; radiographers; radiologists

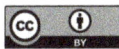

1. Introduction

Artificial intelligence (AI) is a broad, umbrella term that encompasses the theory and development of computer systems able to perform tasks normally requiring human intelligence [1]. In several fields including healthcare, AI is moving quickly from an experimental phase to an implementation phase [2]. The word "AI" includes the sciences and innovations that use computers to simulate, expand, or even enhance human intelligence. AI is directly related to the information technological revolution, cognitive science, analytics, and algorithms [3]. In the best-case scenario, AI algorithms will provide an additional tool for radiologists, close to a "second pair of eyes", giving an additional point of view on cases and improving competency and diagnostic reliability. This is the equivalent of a radiologist asking a colleague whom he or she trusts for a second point of view about a case [4]. In addition, the implementation of AI in medical imaging needs radiological technologists to further adapt with the integration between AI and medical imaging. Therefore, treatment practice and imaging should be enhanced with new technology, as high-quality practice and research will provide benefits to patients [5].

In regard to the imaging reports, there is specialized terminology to describe radiographic appearances precisely, which radiologists share with others within their profession, as well as with referring physicians and patients. As AI technology expands and ultimately becomes a part of the clinical workflow, radiologists need to familiarize themselves with its basic principles and terminology [6]. Medicine and, more specifically, radiology are witnessing continuous changes associated with AI and machine learning [7]. Recently, AI technologies for radiology applications have gained popularity among healthcare providers [8], due to the fact that radiology is one of the most prolific generators of a huge amount of digital data [9], leading to increased work pressures for specialists and radiologists. Therefore, there is a growing need to develop technologies that carry some of the workload [10].

Extensive research has shown that AI technology assists with image recognition and acquisition, improves the support tools for radiology decisions, helps monitor possible diagnostic errors, and facilitates intelligent scheduling solutions [7,11]. The first step toward enhancing the application of AI in radiology requires a deep knowledge of current capabilities and future concerns [12]. However, the radiology community needs to be trained about how to critically analyze the possibilities, risks, and threats associated with the implementation of new AI instruments [2]. In all of the studies reviewed here, no progress could be made in applications of AI related to radiology and medical imaging in Saudi Arabia without surveying the readiness of the workforce in radiology. The role of radiologists in the AI era is to become expert consumers of AI algorithms. There are opportunities to capitalize on the latest emphasis and excitement surrounding modern AI technologies and chances to use data to educate radiologists about their possibilities. The revolution of AI growth is gaining momentum, and the variety of AI applications being presented to radiologists is growing, providing challenges to radiologists about the best tools to select [4].

The most beneficial AI tools for radiologists are the applications that will best fulfil their clinical needs and help them to answer the questions asked by their referring physicians [3]. The radiologists' practice may be enhanced using AI tools, which may affect the their clinical experience [4]. Focusing on the radiologists' knowledge and training on the use of the AI tools is very important, as this assists their practice, which, in turn, benefits patients [4]. Radiologists should collaborate with the computer science and engineering departments of their respective universities and contribute to the research and development of AI in healthcare systems to guarantee that there is full clinical value to the problems under examination [2].

Moreover, there are many areas in medical imaging that show the direct impact of AI on the radiographers' role, such as pre-examination assessment, examination planning, imaging acquisition, and image processing. For example, radiographers usually contact patients directly before imaging to explain the procedures and take care of them after imaging. This is unlikely to be changed by AI technologies. However, there is the potential for AI to contribute to and help in the automated examinations of referrals, checking the clinical indications and confirming the patient's identification via an interface with the Electronic Health Record. AI technologies can also assist in imaging modality techniques and processes [13].

Currently, there are no data to measure the amount of awareness about AI in Saudi Arabia. To address this issue, we performed an electronic survey to assess the radiology community's attitude toward AI applications in Saudi Arabia. This would improve our knowledge on the future direction of choosing radiology as a lifetime career.

2. Materials and Methods

Data for this study were collected using an electronic questionnaire using the Google Forms application, and the link was distributed across Saudi Arabia through emails, WhatsApp groups, and Twitter during the period from 2019 and 2020. A total of 714 participants were included in the study. The target group in this study was radiologists, radiology technologists, technicians, and radiological sciences students from different regions around Saudi Arabia. The questionnaire consisted of two parts. The first part was related to demographic data that contained gender, age, highest qualification attained, and subspecialty. The second part was structured into eight sections with a total of 25 statements. Each section addressed different aspects of AI technology (see Appendix). The first section contained questions on the participants' awareness of AI, and section two covered AI applications in clinical practice. Sections three to five dealt with AI results, AI responsibilities, and AI validation, respectively. Section six focused on the role of the patient, whereas section seven focused on the benefits of AI in medicine. The last section was related to the future of AI.

A three-point Likert scale was used, and the participants were asked to answer each question using one of the following options: (Agree, Neutral, Disagree). To simplify the analysis, the neutral responses were considered negative and ultimately were regarded as a disagreement with the question. Data management and analysis were performed using SPSS Statistics (version 25). This study did not require ethical approval because there was no risk to the participants. A one-way ANOVA and chi square were used to compare the differences in the awareness of the participants. When there was no homogeneity of variance, and in order to minimize Type 1 error, the more conservative Welch's *t*-test was applied.

3. Results

3.1. Descriptive Data Analysis

A total of 714 individuals participated in the study. Of them, 45.4% (N = 324) were female and 54.6% (N = 390) were male. The age distribution of participants is shown in Figure 1. The inclusion of participants with varying age allowed for the assessment of differing experiences of individuals, as experience might change with age. The majority of participants (n = 245; 34%) belonged to the age range of 20 to 25 years. This was followed by participants belonging to the age range of 26 to 30 years (n = 172; 24%), 31 to 35 years (n = 123; 17%), and more than 40 years (n = 83; 12%).

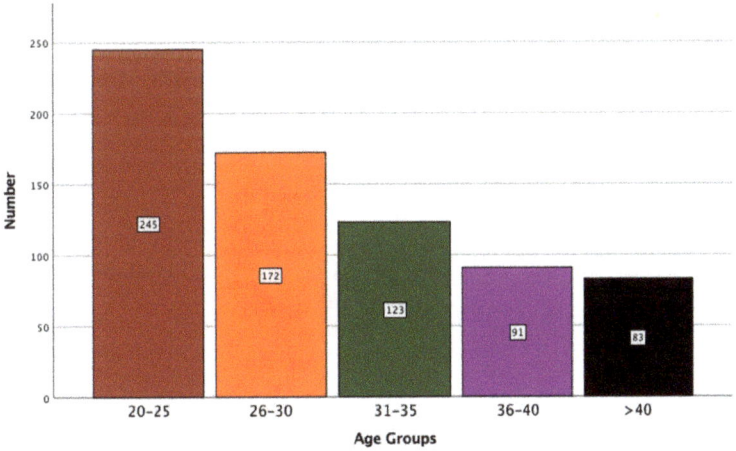

Figure 1. A bar graph showing the distribution of participants based on their age.

In the present study, the qualifications of the participants were distributed by a breakdown of 44.7% (N = 319) with a bachelor's degree, 6.9% (N = 49) with a diploma, 15% (N = 107) with a masters, 14.6% (N = 104) with a Ph.D., and 135 (18.9%) of them were undergraduate students. Through the inclusion of participants with different educational levels, the relevant attitudes could be understood. The participants' profession and locations are graphically represented in Figures 2 and 3, respectively.

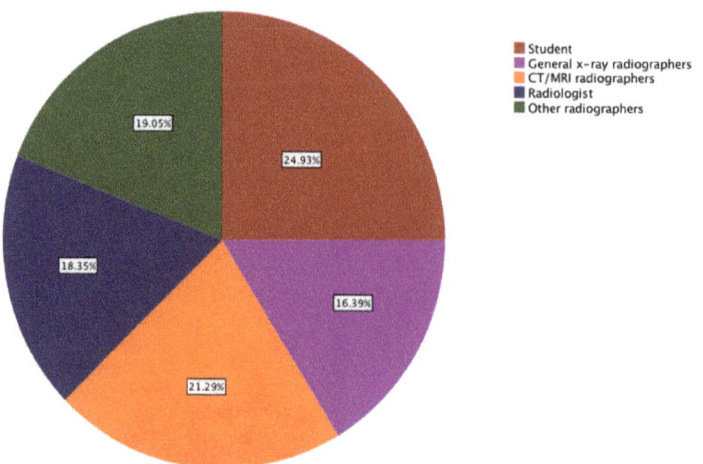

Figure 2. A pie graph showing the distribution of participants based on their professions.

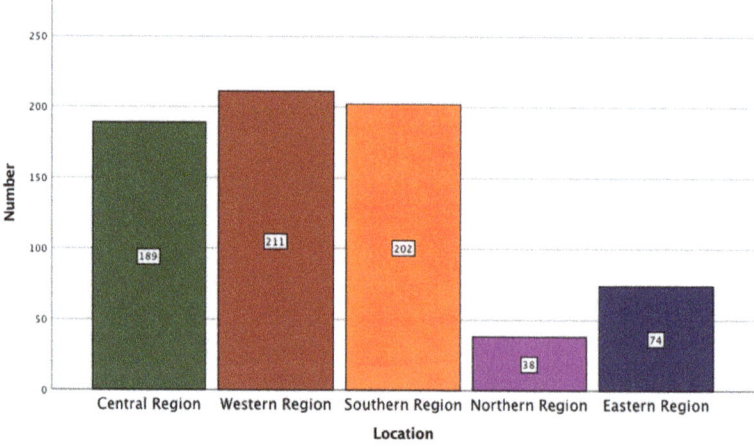

Figure 3. A bar graph showing the distribution of participants based on their locations.

3.2. AI Awareness

The first set of questions aimed to evaluate the participants' awareness of AI in general, and its uses in radiology in particular (Table 1). It is clear from Table 1 that the majority of the participants (61.2%) have read or heard about the role of AI in radiology. Interestingly, the odds of male participants reading or hearing about the role of AI in radiology is significantly higher than that for female participants (odd ratio (OR): 2.4, 95% confidence interval (CI): 1.76 to 3.3, $p < 0.001$). Moreover, participants who are more than 30 years of age are more likely to have read or heard about AI in radiology (OR: 0.47, CI: 0.34 to 0.64, $p < 0.001$). In addition, there was a significant difference between the group means according to their education level as determined by one-way ANOVA (Welch's $F (2, 426.7) = 46.4$, $p < 0.005$). From this, we can infer that participants with a high level of education are more likely to have read or heard about AI. We also observed that radiologists have statistically different responses and tend to read more about AI compared to all other professions, (Welch's $F (4, 709) = 24$, $p < 0.005$).

Table 1. Awareness responses.

Questions	Answers	No.	%
Have you ever read or heard about artificial intelligence and its role in radiology?	Agree	437	61.2
	Disagree	277	38.8
Is your knowledge about artificial intelligence based on what is published in the media?	Agree	453	63.4
	Disagree	261	36.6
Are you keen to attend conferences and courses about artificial intelligence in radiology?	Agree	311	43.6
	Disagree	403	56.4
Are you involved in research projects on developing applications of artificial intelligence?	Agree	170	23.8
	Disagree	544	76.2
Does artificial intelligence contribute in the preparation of radiographic reports?	Agree	389	54.5
	Disagree	325	45.5

In addition, less than half the participants (44%) were keen to attend conferences or courses about AI in radiology. A closer inspection showed that the females as well as younger participants were less likely to attend conferences compared with the males and the older group, (OR: 1.6, CI: 1.2 to 2.2, $p < 0.005$ and OR: 0.4, CI: 0.33 to 0.6, $p < 0.001$, respectively). Surprisingly, participants who specialized in CT/MRI were more eager to attend conferences than radiologists were, (Welch's $F(4, 341) = 9.4$, $p < 0.001$).

Moreover, male and older groups were almost twice as more likely to be involved in research involving AI compared with the female and younger groups, (OR: 2, CI: 1.4 to 2.0, $p < 0.001$, OR: 0.55, CI: 0.39 to 0.8, $p < 0.005$, respectively). In addition, we found no significant association between the profession and location in regard to the knowledge about the contribution of AI in the preparation of radiographic reports, $p > 0.05$.

3.3. AI Practices

The second set of questions assessed the participants' knowledge of the practices of AI in radiology (Table 2). The results showed that the vast majority of people (71.3%) agreed with the statement that AI contributed to the capture of high-quality images. Our statistical analysis showed that both the gender and age had no effect on the participants' decision on this question, $p > 0.5$. Furthermore, radiologists significantly differed from college students in that they were more likely to disagree with the use of AI in the selection of scanning protocols for CT and MRI, $p < 0.05$. Interestingly, although the majority of participants believed that AI could help in obtaining high-quality images and assist with the archiving system, only about half felt that their jobs were threatened by this technology. What was interesting about the data in this table was that the participants' education levels and locations did not appear to have an effect on their responses.

Table 2. Awareness responses.

Questions	Answers	No.	%
Artificial intelligence contributes to obtain high-quality images	Agree	509	71.3
	Disagree	205	28.7
Artificial intelligence contributes to the archiving system (PACS)	Agree	576	80.7
	Disagree	138	19.3
Artificial intelligence contributes toward the selection of appropriate scanning protocols for CT/MRI imaging	Agree	456	63.9
	Disagree	258	36.1
Is the weakness in training new graduates on artificial intelligence skills one of the greatest obstacles to the application of artificial intelligence in the work environment?	Agree	493	69
	Disagree	221	31
Will the application of artificial intelligence threaten some radiological professions?	Agree	312	43.7
	Disagree	402	56.3

3.4. AI Outcomes

The third set of questions assessed the participants' knowledge of the outcomes of AI in radiology (Table 3). Closer inspection of Table 3 showed that 60% of the participants felt the results produced by AI are not reliable. The belief was more common in B.Sc. holders and higher education levels compared with that in diploma holders and college students, (Welch's F (2, 717.9) = 7.67, $p < 0.01$). Even though 80% of the participants thought that the results produced by AI should be verified by radiologists, this was found to be significant between the participating radiologists and other professionals, (Welch's F (4, 434.4) = 8.02, $p < 0.001$). When the participants were asked about whether AI causes stress and anxiety to the patients, 60% of them agreed. Further analysis showed that the younger group were more likely to agree with this statement, (OR: 1.9, CI: 1 to 1.9, $p < 0.05$). Finally, the majority of participants thought that radiologists should not have to bear the responsibility of the results obtained by utilizing AI but that it should be shared between AI companies and organizations, 75% and 83%, respectively.

Table 3. Outcomes responses.

Questions	Answers	No.	%
Can the result of radiographic examination by the artificial intelligence be considered reliable in routine cases?	Agree	285	39.9
	Disagree	429	60.1
The results of radiographic examination by the artificial intelligence need to be verified by the radiologist	Agree	568	79.6
	Disagree	146	20.4
Does conflict in results and interpretation between the various artificial intelligence algorithms and the opinion of the doctor cause stress and anxiety for the patient	Agree	425	59.5
	Disagree	289	40.5
The radiologists are the only ones responsible for the results of the utilization of artificial intelligence	Agree	182	25.5
	Disagree	532	74.5
Shared responsibility must be applied between artificial intelligence companies, hospitals, and international organizations regarding the results of using of artificial intelligence	Agree	595	83.3
	Disagree	119	16.7

3.5. AI Responsibilities

The fourth set of questions assessed the participants' knowledge of the responsibilities of AI in radiology (Table 4). It was apparent from this table that 88% of the participants agreed with having the results verified before they were approved. Interestingly, radiographers in the X-ray department were more likely to answer differently compared with the CT/MRI staff and radiologists, (Welch's F (4, 342) = 4.54, $p = 0.001$). Of the study population, 65% agreed that patients should be aware of using AI, and their consent should be obtained. Younger participants were more likely to agree with this compared with their older counterparts (OR: 1.5, CI: 1.1 to 2, $p < 0.05$). When patients were asked about whether AI contributes to the quality of patient care, only 61% agreed. Further analysis of this question revealed that the males and the older group were more likely to agree with this statement compared with the females and the younger group, (OR: 1.5, CI: 1.1 to 2, $p < 0.05$ and OR: 0.6, CI: 0.46 to 0.85, $p < 0.05$, respectively). Similarly, 62% of the participants thought AI could make radiologists and physicians more efficient in their practice and the males and the older group were more likely to agree, (OR: 1.5, CI: 1.1 to 2, $p < 0.05$ and OR: 0.6, CI: 0.4 to 0.77, $p < 0.001$, respectively).

Table 4. Responsibilities responses.

Questions	Answers	No.	%
The validity of the results from artificial intelligence must be verified	Agree	628	88
	Disagree	86	12
The patient should be aware of the use of artificial intelligence, and his or her consent should be obtained	Agree	463	64.8
	Disagree	251	35.2
The use of artificial intelligence contributes to the improvement of patient care	Agree	437	61.2
	Disagree	277	38.8
Should information issued about artificial intelligence be available only to radiologists?	Agree	238	33.3
	Disagree	476	66.7
Does the use of artificial intelligence enhance the capabilities of both physicians and radiologists and make them more efficient?	Agree	445	62.3
	Disagree	269	37.7

3.6. AI Validation

The final set of questions assessed the participants' knowledge on the validation of AI in radiology (Table 5). Of the 714 participants, 65% of them felt that the use of AI made medical services more accurate. Further analysis showed that the older group were more likely to agree with this statement, (OR: 0.7, CI: 0.52 to 1, $p < 0.05$). Moreover, the majority of the participants (74%) did not think the use of AI made the medical services more humane. Male respondents compared to their counterparts were almost twice more likely to agree with this, (OR: 1.7, CI: 1.2 to 2.4, $p < 0.05$). In addition, 82% of the participants felt that AI must be included in the curriculum of medical and allied health colleges. In addition, 86% of the participants agreed that AI would be essential in the future. Further analysis showed that the responses of the participants from the eastern region were significantly different from those of their counterparts from the southern region, (Welch's F (4, 191.8) = 4.7, $p = 0.001$). Even though the interaction between machine and men would be one of the most important skills in the future, 89% of the participants thought that it would never replace radiologists.

Table 5. Validation responses.

Questions	Answers	No.	%
The use of artificial intelligence makes medical services more accurate	Agree	463	64.8
	Disagree	251	35.2
The use of artificial intelligence makes medical services more humane	Agree	189	26.5
	Disagree	525	73.5
Artificial intelligence must be included in the curriculum and training of medicine and health sciences colleges	Agree	585	81.9
	Disagree	129	18.1
Artificial intelligence cannot dispense with the role of physician and radiologist but makes a change in the work environment	Agree	635	88.9
	Disagree	79	11.1
The interaction between man and machine will be one of the most important medical skills in the future.	Agree	617	86.4
	Disagree	97	13.6

4. Discussion

AI can significantly improve the performance of healthcare providers. This is vital in radiology since radiology is one of the largest generators of big data. The transformation to AI can assist in reducing the workload of healthcare providers as well as improving image acquisition and evaluation. However, there is a lack of studies on how radiology specialists and radiologists would perceive such a transformation, particularly in Saudi Arabia. To our knowledge, this is the first publication of this kind to include all radiology staff from all over Saudi Arabia.

The findings presented in this study showed that the majority of the participants have read or heard about AI, mainly through the media (63%). The study confirmed that the media played an important role in shaping public perception. These results reflected those of Goldberg et al., who also found that the media characterized public perspectives regarding the use of AI in radiology [14]. Approximately 60% of our sample claimed that treatment was made more effective by using AI. This is consistent with the analysis by Gong et al., in which more than 90% of Canadian medical students accepted that AI would improve the potential of radiologists and make them more effective [15].

In our research, 80% of the respondents agreed that AI technologies must be validated in a well-established clinical setting. The medical societies had to address concerns about how to test AI software for therapeutic efficacy and safety prior to the implementation of a large AI clinical application [16]. Various investigations examined and contrasted AI resources to extremely advanced activities, such as X-ray pneumonia diagnosis or mammogram breast cancer screening [17]. However, these algorithms were constrained in some anatomical regions to particular diseases. Nowadays, the superiority of computers over humans is not a matter of debate; rather, the question is centered around how the practice of medicine can benefit from these capabilities [18]. The detection of pulmonary nodules and wrist fractures has been shown to be enhanced by the use of AI [19–21]. Nevertheless, this may lead to a concern in regard to biasing the physician's decision [22].

In addition, we identified differences between the attitudes of the radiology staff concerning the securing the patient's approval prior to the use of AI. They all agreed with the statement that patients should be informed. Because discrepancies between the evaluation of radiologists and AI could lead to patients' irritation and doubt, this question is still one of the key areas concerning the use of AI in radiology [16]. Moreover, 82% of the respondents stated that AI should be integrated into the medical curricula. This is consistent with a study by Dos Santos et al., where 77% believed that AI will revolutionize radiology and should be included in medical education [23,24].

Gong et al. showed that about 30% of medical students think that AI will replace radiologists in the future [15]. This differed against the findings presented in this study, where only 11% collectively shared this opinion. There were similarities between the attitudes expressed by the participants in this study and those described by Dos Santos et al., where 83% of the respondents disagreed with the statement that AI would replace human radiologists [23]. Another recently published study found that radiologists have a positive attitude toward the implementation of AI and are not concerned that AI will replace them [25]. At the same time, AI may replace human medical expertise in specific and repetitive tasks, such as detecting disease indicators in images [26]. Finally, the majority of the participants (84%) agreed with the fact that the interaction between man and machine is one of the most important skills in the future. This is consistent with the findings of Davenport and Kalakota, who showed that only those who refused to work alongside AI will lose their jobs [27].

5. Conclusions

This study is the first Saudi survey to assess the awareness and attitude of the radiology community in regard to AI applications. Because AI plays a role in image recognition and acquisition and also improves the support tools for radiology decisions, it is important to ensure that radiologists and radiographers have at least a minimum understanding of the technology. Our finding demonstrated the participants possessed an acceptable level of knowledge regarding AI technology. It also showed that the interaction between man and machine would be one of the most important skills in the future, and thus, AI applications should be included in the curriculum of medical students. A natural progression of this work is to analyze the impact of AI on routine radiology procedures and the challenges facing its clinical implementation in Saudi Arabia.

Author Contributions: Conceptualization, M.A., M.S.A., F.A., N.A., and H.A.; methodology, S.A. (Sultan Alamri) and A.M.; validation, M.A. and S.A. (Salem Alelyani); formal analysis, M.S.A., N.A.

and F.A.; writing—review and editing, M.A., S.A. (Sultan Alamri) and H.A.; supervision, A.M. and S.A. (Salem Alelyani). All authors have read and agreed to the published version of the manuscript.

Funding: The authors extend their appreciation for funds provided by the Deanship of Scientific Research at King Khalid University through grant number (R.G.P2/100/41).

Institutional Review Board Statement: The study was conducted according to the guidelines of the Declaration of Helsinki and approved by the Ethics Committee at King Khaled University on 9 November 2020.

Informed Consent Statement: Not applicable.

Acknowledgments: We deeply acknowledge Taif University for supporting the researchers through Taif University Researchers Supporting Project number (TURSP-2020/287), Taif University, Taif, Saudi Arabia.

Conflicts of Interest: The authors declare no conflict of interest.

References

1. Reyes, M.; Meier, R.; Pereira, S.; Silva, C.A.; Dahlweid, F.-M.; von Tengg-Kobligk, H.; Summers, R.M.; Wiest, R. On the Interpretability of Artificial Intelligence in Radiology: Challenges and Opportunities. *Radiol. Artif. Intell.* **2020**, *2*, e190043. [CrossRef] [PubMed]
2. Tang, A.; Tam, R.; Cadrin-Chênevert, A.; Guest, W.; Chong, J.; Barfett, J.; Chepelev, L.; Cairns, R.; Mitchell, J.R.; Cicero, M.D.; et al. Canadian Association of Radiologists White Paper on Artificial Intelligence in Radiology. *Can. Assoc. Radiol. J.* **2018**, *69*, 120–135. [CrossRef] [PubMed]
3. SFR-IA Group; Cerf; French Radiology Community. Artificial intelligence and medical imaging 2018: French Radiology Community white paper. *Diagn. Interv. Imaging* **2018**, *99*, 727–742. [CrossRef]
4. Rubin, D.L. Artificial Intelligence in Imaging: The Radiologist's Role. *J. Am. Coll. Radiol.* **2019**, *16*, 1309–1317. [CrossRef]
5. International Society of Radiographers and Radiological Technologists; The European Federation Of Radiographer Societies. Artificial Intelligence and the Radiographer/Radiological Technologist Profession: A joint statement of the International Society of Radiographers and Radiological Technologists and the European Federation of Radiographer Societies. *Radiography* **2020**, *26*, 93–95. [CrossRef]
6. Minka, T. A Statistical Learning/Pattern Recognition Glossary. 2006. Available online: http://alumni.media.mit.edu/~{}tpminka/statlearn/glossary/ (accessed on 21 March 2021).
7. Ranschaert, E.R.; Morozov, S.; Algra, P.R. (Eds.) *Artificial Intelligence in Medical Imaging: Opportunities, Applications and Risks*; Springer International Publishing: Berlin/Heidelberg, Germany, 2019. [CrossRef]
8. Topol, E.J. High-performance medicine: The convergence of human and artificial intelligence. *Nat. Med.* **2019**, *25*, 44–56. [CrossRef]
9. European Society of Radiology (ESR). Impact of artificial intelligence on radiology: A EuroAIM survey among members of the European Society of Radiology. *Insights Imaging* **2019**, *10*, 105. [CrossRef]
10. Liu, X.; Faes, L.; Kale, A.U.; Wagner, S.K.; Fu, D.J.; Bruynseels, A.; Mahendiran, T.; Moraes, G.; Shamdas, M.; Kern, C.; et al. A comparison of deep learning performance against health-care professionals in detecting diseases from medical imaging: A systematic review and meta-analysis. *Lancet Digit. Health* **2019**, *1*, e271–e297. [CrossRef]
11. Choy, G.; Khalilzadeh, O.; Michalski, M.; Synho, D.; Samir, A.E.; Pianykh, O.S.; Geis, J.R.; Pandharipande, P.V.; Brink, J.A.; Dreyer, K.J. Current Applications and Future Impact of Machine Learning in Radiology. *Radiology* **2018**, *288*, 318–328. [CrossRef] [PubMed]
12. Liew, C. The future of radiology augmented with Artificial Intelligence: A strategy for success. *Eur. J. Radiol.* **2018**, *102*, 152–156. [CrossRef] [PubMed]
13. Hardy, M.; Harvey, H. Artificial intelligence in diagnostic imaging: Impact on the radiography profession. *Br. J. Radiol.* **2020**, *93*, 20190840. [CrossRef]
14. Goldberg, J.E.; Rosenkrantz, A. Artificial Intelligence and Radiology: A Social Media Perspective. *Curr. Probl. Diagn. Radiol.* **2019**, *48*, 308–311. [CrossRef]
15. Gong, B.; Nugent, J.P.; Guest, W.; Parker, W.; Chang, P.J.; Khosa, F.; Nicolaou, S. Influence of Artificial Intelligence on Canadian Medical Students' Preference for Radiology Specialty: ANational Survey Study. *Acad. Radiol.* **2019**, *26*, 566–577. [CrossRef]
16. Geis, J.R.; Brady, A.; Wu, C.C.; Spencer, J.; Ranschaert, E.; Jaremko, J.L.; Langer, S.G.; Kitts, A.B.; Birch, J.; Shields, W.F.; et al. Ethics of artificial intelligence in radiology: Summary of the joint European and North American multisociety statement. *Insights Imaging* **2019**, *10*, 101. [CrossRef]
17. McKinney, S.M.; Sieniek, M.; Godbole, V.; Godwin, J.; Antropova, N.; Ashrafian, H.; Back, T.; Chesus, M.; Corrado, G.S.; Darzi, A.; et al. International evaluation of an AI system for breast cancer screening. *Nature* **2020**, *577*, 89–94. [CrossRef] [PubMed]
18. Celi, L.A.; Fine, B.; Stone, D.J. An awakening in medicine: The partnership of humanity and intelligent machines. *Lancet Digit. Health* **2019**, *1*, e255–e257. [CrossRef]

19. Nam, J.G.; Park, S.; Hwang, E.J.; Lee, J.H.; Jin, K.-N.; Lim, K.Y.; Vu, T.H.; Sohn, J.H.; Hwang, S.; Goo, J.M.; et al. Development and Validation of Deep Learning–based Automatic Detection Algorithm for Malignant Pulmonary Nodules on Chest Radiographs. *Radiology* **2019**, *290*, 218–228. [CrossRef]
20. Lindsey, R.; Daluiski, A.; Chopra, S.; Lachapelle, A.; Mozer, M.; Sicular, S.; Hanel, D.; Gardner, M.; Gupta, A.; Hotchkiss, R.; et al. Deep neural network improves fracture detection by clinicians. *Proc. Natl. Acad. Sci. USA* **2018**, *115*, 11591–11596. [CrossRef]
21. Blanc, D.; Racine, V.; Khalil, A.; Deloche, M.; Broyelle, J.-A.; Hammouamri, I.; Sinitambirivoutin, E.; Fiammante, M.; Verdier, E.; Besson, T.; et al. Artificial intelligence solution to classify pulmonary nodules on CT. *Diagn. Interv. Imaging* **2020**, *101*, 803–810. [CrossRef]
22. Uyumazturk, B.; Kiani, A.; Rajpurkar, P.; Wang, A.; Ball, R.L.; Gao, R.; Yu, Y.; Jones, E.; Langlotz, C.P.; Martin, B.; et al. Deep Learning for the Digital Pathologic Diagnosis of Cholangiocarcinoma and Hepatocellular Carcinoma: Evaluating the Impact of a Web-based Diagnostic Assistant. *arXiv* **2019**, arXiv:1911.07372.
23. Dos Santos, D.P.; Giese, D.; Brodehl, S.; Chon, S.-H.; Staab, W.; Kleinert, R.; Maintz, D.; Baeßler, B. Medical students' attitude towards artificial intelligence: A multicentre survey. *Eur. Radiol.* **2019**, *29*, 1640–1646. [CrossRef] [PubMed]
24. Huisman, M.; Ranschaert, E.; Parker, W.; Mastrodicasa, D.; Koci, M.; de Santos, D.P.; Coppola, F.; Morozov, S.; Zins, M.; Bohyn, C.; et al. An international survey on AI in radiology in 1,041 radiologists and radiology residents part 1: Fear of replacement, knowledge, and attitude. *Eur. Radiol.* **2021**. [CrossRef] [PubMed]
25. Coppola, F.; Faggioni, L.; Regge, D.; Giovagnoni, A.; Golfieri, R.; Bibbolino, C.; Miele, V.; Neri, E.; Grassi, R. Artificial intelligence: Radiologists' expectations and opinions gleaned from a nationwide online survey. *Radiol. Med.* **2021**, *126*, 63–71. [CrossRef]
26. Savadjiev, P.; Chong, J.; Dohan, A.; Vakalopoulou, M.; Reinhold, C.; Paragios, N.; Gallix, B. Demystification of AI-driven medical image interpretation: Past, present and future. *Eur. Radiol.* **2019**, *29*, 1616–1624. [CrossRef] [PubMed]
27. Davenport, T.; Kalakota, R. The potential for artificial intelligence in healthcare. *Future Healthc. J.* **2019**, *6*, 94–98. [CrossRef] [PubMed]

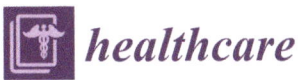

Article

Role of Artificial Intelligence Interpretation of Colposcopic Images in Cervical Cancer Screening

Seongmin Kim [1], Hwajung Lee [2], Sanghoon Lee [2], Jae-Yun Song [2,*], Jae-Kwan Lee [2] and Nak-Woo Lee [2]

[1] Gynecologic Cancer Center, CHA Ilsan Medical Center, CHA University College of Medicine, 1205 Jungang-ro, Ilsandong-gu, Goyang-si 10414, Korea; naiad515@gmail.com

[2] Department of Obstetrics and Gynecology, Korea University College of Medicine, 73 Inchon-ro, Seongbuk-gu, Seoul 02841, Korea; ifigured35@gmail.com (H.L.); mdleesh@gmail.com (S.L.); jklee38@korea.ac.kr (J.-K.L.); nwlee@korea.ac.kr (N.-W.L.)

* Correspondence: yuni105@korea.ac.kr; Tel.: +82-2-920-6775

Abstract: The accuracy of colposcopic diagnosis depends on the skill and proficiency of physicians. This study evaluated the feasibility of interpreting colposcopic images with the assistance of artificial intelligence (AI) for the diagnosis of high-grade cervical intraepithelial lesions. This study included female patients who underwent colposcopy-guided biopsy in 2020 at two institutions in the Republic of Korea. Two experienced colposcopists reviewed all images separately. The Cerviray AI® system (AIDOT, Seoul, Korea) was used to interpret the cervical images. AI demonstrated improved sensitivity with comparable specificity and positive predictive value when compared with the colposcopic impressions of each clinician. The areas under the curve were greater with combined impressions (both AI and that of the two colposcopists) of high-grade lesions, when compared with the individual impressions of each colposcopist. This study highlights the feasibility of the application of an AI system in cervical cancer screening. AI interpretation can be utilized as an assisting tool in combination with human colposcopic evaluation of exocervix.

Keywords: artificial intelligence; cervical cancer screening; colposcopy; deep learning; machine learning

1. Introduction

Cervical intraepithelial neoplasia (CIN) is a premalignant lesion that is diagnosed and categorized as CIN1, CIN2, or CIN3 [1]. Genital human papillomavirus (HPV) infection is known as the critical step in the development of CIN [2]. If CIN is untreated, some patients may develop cervical cancer [3]. A diagnosis of CIN2-3 is a histological diagnosis obtained from biopsies of the suspect lesions, either with or without colposcopy, for which treatment is recommended. Screening for CIN can be achieved by cytological examination, human papillomavirus (HPV) screening, or colposcopy [4]. Among these, primary HPV testing is the most preferred method globally [5]. Regular screening for cervical cancer may lower the lifetime risk of the disease [6]. However, screening programs in low-income countries are difficult due to inaccessibility, lack of funding, lack of public policies, and high costs [7].

Colposcopy is used to identify cervical lesions using low-magnification microscopy with acetic acid and Lugol's solution. It carries a sensitivity of 66–96% and specificity of 35–98% in diagnosing cervical lesions [8–10]. However, its accuracy varies according to the physician's skill or proficiency [11].

The use of artificial intelligence (AI) in the medical field can improve the quality of care and cost-effectiveness [12]. Although machine learning can process a large amount of data in a relatively short time and has been successfully applied in many clinical situations, effective utilization of machine learning in actual clinical practice remains difficult [13]. Several studies have demonstrated the feasibility of clinical applications of AI in improving the diagnostic quality in CIN [14–17]. Previous studies evaluated the diagnostic value of AI for the interpretation of cervical images compared to that of cytology or histology.

The purpose of this study was to evaluate the feasibility of an AI system as an assistant tool in diagnosing high-grade CIN lesions compared to human interpretation of cervical images.

2. Materials and Methods

2.1. Study Patients and Terminology

This study included female patients who underwent colposcopy-guided biopsy because of abnormal cervical cytology or a positive HPV status during 2020 at two institutions located in Goyang and Seoul, Korea. Patients younger than 20 years or older than 50 years were excluded from the study. Additionally, unsatisfactory colposcopic images because of poor focus or invisible transformational zone were excluded from the study. Patient data along with cytologic and histopathological results following the biopsy were required for inclusion in the study. The cytological results in the data include either conventional Pap smear or liquid-based cytology. The histological results were obtained from the pathologic report from the biopsy, which was diagnosed by a professional pathologist in both institutions. Colposcopic images only included the cervical images with acetic acid applied on the cervix; images with Lugol's solution applied on the cervix were not included. This study was approved by the institutional review board (2019AN0019). Bethesda classification system and CIN classification system were used for cytologic and histologic evaluation, respectively. The International Federation for Cervical Pathology and Colposcopy terminology was used for determining colposcopic impression.

2.2. Preparation of Machine Learning System

To interpret the cervical imaging, the Cerviray AI® machine learning system (AIDOT, Seoul, Korea) was used, constructed with over 10,000 colposcopic images that were introduced to the learning algorithm along with histopathological diagnoses and clinical impressions of three gynecologic experts in colposcopy. A multi-category deep learning method was used by integrating (1) a knowledge-based clinical decision support system (CDSS) using the clinical colposcopic findings and histopathological results, and (2) non-knowledge-based CDSS via machine learning. The results interpreted by AI were classified as normal, CIN1, CIN2-3, or cancer. Figure 1 illustrates the interpretation of images using Cerviray AI® deep learning system, which is composed of three main modules as follows:

(1) Satisfactory filtering module was introduced to differentiate whether the taken colposcopic image is adequately satisfied for screening. This module is implemented by a convolutional neural network (CNN)-based classification model, which was trained to yield binary results that consist of satisfactory and unsatisfactory.

(2) Preprocessing and normalization module was applied to prepare and adjust the image before AI interpretation. Colposcopic images are usually captured in uncontrolled environments, which result in various quality of the taken images such as poor contrast, brightness, etc. To compensate and improve the quality of the images, an auto-adjustment algorithm was implemented to preprocess and normalize them by applying various thresholding and filtering methods.

(3) Feature extraction and cervical cancer diagnosis module have an important role in exploring the regions of the colposcopic images which correspond to suspicious precancerous cervical lesions. This module is implemented by CNN-based multi-class detection model named AIDOTNet v1.2, which was trained with multi-category images that consists the location of low and high-grade lesions. AIDOTNet v1.2 utilizes a pre-trained model to extract the suspicious region from a given image for predicting the lesion location in the image. In other words, the model leverages the feature extraction from the pre-trained model to locate the suspicious lesion box in the image and finally classifies the detected box as CIN1, CIN2-3, or cancer lesion. However, if no suspicious lesion box is detected from the colposcopic image, the model will yield normal as the AI interpretation result.

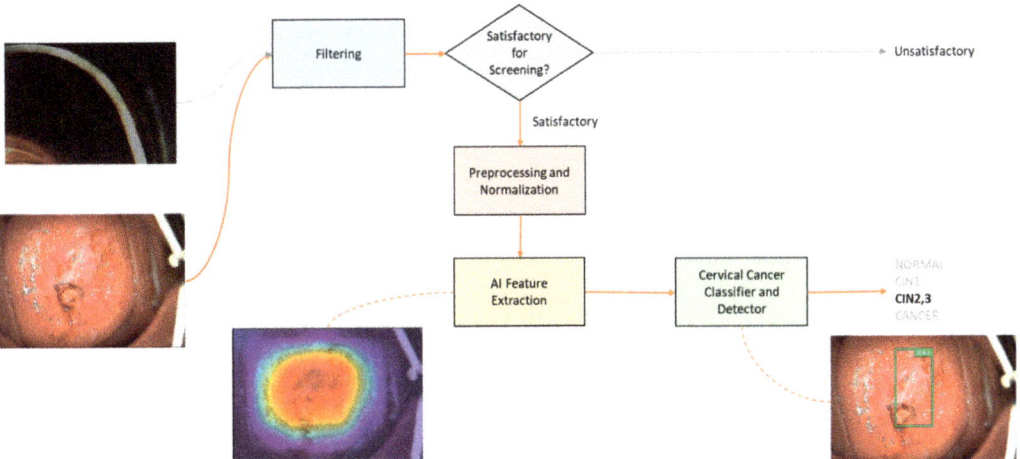

Figure 1. A diagram of Cerviray AI® interpretation for colposcopic images. The system assesses the visibility of the images, and recognizes the squamocolumnar junction and transformation zone of the uterine cervix. If the image is satisfactory for evaluation, the image is processed and normalized for AI feature extraction. This is followed by the classification of images according to the AI impression.

2.3. Clinical Interpretation of Colposcopic Finding

Two gynecologic oncologists separately examined all the images. Colposcopic impressions were divided into "non-specific", "minor", "major", or "suspicious for invasion". Multiple images of each patient were evaluated for an accurate diagnosis.

2.4. Statistical Analysis

Statistical analysis was performed using SPSS version 22.0 (IBM Inc., Armonk, NY, USA). The Kolmogorov–Smirnov test was used to verify the assumptions of the standard normal distributions. The Student's t-test and Mann–Whitney U test were used to analyze the parametric and non-parametric variables, respectively. Differences between proportions were compared using Fisher's exact test or χ^2 test. Statistical significance was set at $p < 0.05$. Diagnostic accuracy was compared in terms of the sensitivity, specificity, and positive predictive value (PPV) between the cytological findings, colposcopic impressions, AI interpretations, and histopathological results. Pearson's correlation coefficient was used to compare the correlations between the diagnostic tools. The accuracy of the diagnoses was evaluated in the validation set using receiver-operating characteristic (ROC) curves, which were created by plotting sensitivity against the false positive rate and its summary statistic, the area under the curve (AUC).

3. Results

3.1. Patient and Disease Characteristics

Overall, 234 patients were included in this study. The characteristics of the study population and diseases are presented in Table 1. Atypical squamous cells of unknown significance (ASC-US) were the commonest cytological result. The most frequent histological diagnosis was CIN2-3 followed by CIN1, benign findings including chronic cervicitis or koilocytotosis, and invasive cervical cancer. Almost half of the patients did not require any treatment; however, most of the patients with high-grade lesions were treated with conization or loop electrosurgical excision procedure (LEEP).

Table 1. Clinical Characteristics of Study Population.

Characteristics	Value
Age, years	36.9 ± 8.9
Cytological results	
Normal	5 (2.1)
ASC-US	107 (45.7)
LSIL	67 (28.6)
ASC-H/HSIL	52 (22.2)
SCC	3 (1.3)
HPV status	
Positive for high-risk	153 (65.4)
Positive for low-risk only or negative	16 (6.8)
Not done	65 (27.8)
Histopathology	
Benign	52 (22.2)
CIN1	66 (28.2)
CIN2-3	110 (47.0)
Invasive cancer	6 (2.6)
Treatment	
Observation and follow-up	111 (47.4)
LEEP/Conization	107 (45.7)
Extrafascial hysterectomy	5 (2.1)
Radical hysterectomy	4 (1.7)
Chemotherapy/Radiotherapy	2 (0.9)
Refusal of treatment	5 (2.1)

Values are expressed as mean ± standard deviation or number (%). ASC-H: atypical squamous cells, cannot exclude high-grade squamous intraepithelial lesions; ASC-US, atypical squamous cells of unknown significance; CIN, cervical intraepithelial neoplasia; HSIL, high-grade squamous intraepithelial lesion; HPV, human papilloma virus; LEEP, loop electrosurgical excision procedure; LSIL, low-grade squamous intraepithelial lesion.

3.2. Evaluation of Diagnostic Accuracy

The distributions of impressions with each diagnostic tool according to the cytologic results are summarized in Table 2. ASC-US cytology resulted in various histological diagnoses, including benign lesion, CIN1, CIN2-3; otherwise, low-grade squamous intraepithelial lesion (LSIL) and high-grade squamous intraepithelial lesion (HSIL) cytology mostly resulted in corresponding histology.

The sensitivity, specificity, and PPV of each diagnostic tool are summarized in Table 3. AI demonstrated improved sensitivity with similar specificity and PPV compared with the colposcopic impression of each clinician. The sensitivity improved when the impressions of the two modalities were combined with at least one tool reporting suspicious high-grade lesions. The specificity of cytology was the highest among the tools compared.

Figure 2 illustrates the ROC curves for each diagnostic performance. AI demonstrated a higher AUC than Doctor 2 and a lower AUC than Doctor 1. However, if impressions of high-grade lesions were combined from the AI system and each Doctor, the AUCs improved compared with those of each clinician's impressions.

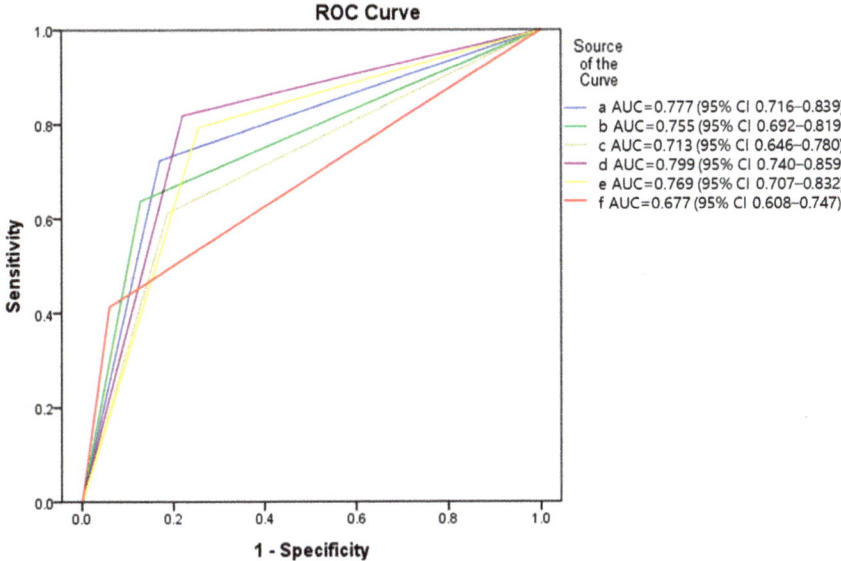

Figure 2. ROC curves of each diagnostic performance for detecting high-grade or worse lesion versus less severe impressions. (a) AI interpretation; (b) colposcopic impression of Dr 1; (c) colposcopic impression of Dr 2; (d) combined impression of AI and Dr1 colposcopy; (e) combined impression of AI and Dr2 colposcopy; (f) cytology.

Table 2. Distribution of the colposcopic findings, AI interpretations, and histopathology according to the cytology results.

Cytology	Impression	Doctor 1	Doctor 2	AI	Histopathology
Normal	Non-specific/Benign	2	2	3	4
	Minor/CIN1	2	3	2	0
	Major/CIN2-3	1	0	0	1
ASC-US	Non-specific/Benign	28	35	43	37
	Minor/CIN1	50	32	30	34
	Major/CIN2-3	32	39	32	35
	Suspicious for invasion/Cancer	0	1	2	1
LSIL	Non-specific/Benign	15	14	20	7
	Minor/CIN1	37	32	24	29
	Major/CIN2-3	15	21	22	31
	Suspicious for invasion/Cancer	0	0	1	0
ASC-H/HSIL	Non-specific/Benign	4	4	7	4
	Minor/CIN1	6	9	5	3
	Major/CIN2-3	41	38	37	43
	Suspicious for invasion/Cancer	1	1	3	2
SCC	Suspicious for invasion/Cancer	3	3	3	3

Values are expressed as a number. AI, artificial intelligence; ASC-H, atypical squamous cells, cannot exclude high-grade squamous intraepithelial lesions; ASC-US, atypical squamous cells of unknown significance; CIN, cervical intraepithelial neoplasia; HSIL, high-grade squamous intraepithelial lesion; LSIL, low-grade squamous intraepithelial lesion; SCC, squamous cell carcinoma.

Table 3. Evaluation of the diagnostic quality of various tools in detecting high-grade or worse lesions versus less severe impressions.

Method	Sensitivity	Specificity	PPV
Cytology	41.38	94.07	87.27
Doctor 1	71.55	87.29	84.69
Doctor 2	69.83	81.36	78.64
AI interpretation	74.14	83.05	81.13
Doctor 1 + AI	84.48	77.97	79.03
Doctor 2 + AI	83.62	74.58	76.38

AI, artificial intelligence; PPV, positive predictive value; Doctor 1 + AI, if Doctor 1 accepted the more aggressive impressions of AI despite disagreements; Doctor 2 + AI, if Doctor 2 accepted the more aggressive impressions of AI despite disagreements.

3.3. Correlation between Diagnostic Performances

Figure 3 presents the correlation coefficients for each diagnostic tool. Doctors 1 and 2 demonstrated the highest correlation coefficients. However, cytology demonstrated a generally low correlation with other diagnostic tools.

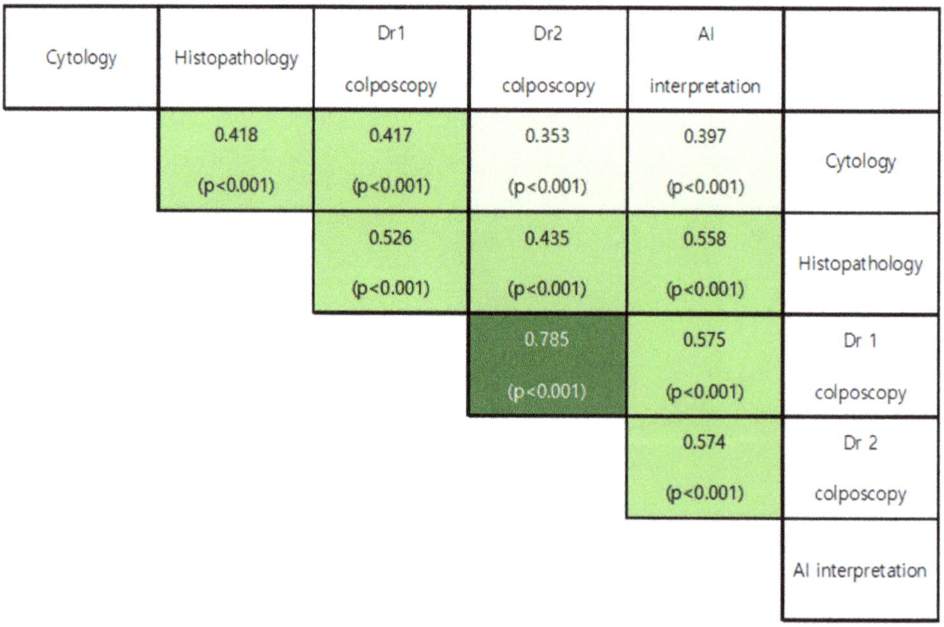

Cytology	Histopathology	Dr1 colposcopy	Dr2 colposcopy	AI interpretation	
	0.418 (p<0.001)	0.417 (p<0.001)	0.353 (p<0.001)	0.397 (p<0.001)	Cytology
		0.526 (p<0.001)	0.435 (p<0.001)	0.558 (p<0.001)	Histopathology
			0.785 (p<0.001)	0.575 (p<0.001)	Dr 1 colposcopy
				0.574 (p<0.001)	Dr 2 colposcopy
					AI interpretation

Figure 3. Correlations between each diagnostic tool. Values are expressed as Pearson's R (*p*-value).

4. Discussion

Colposcopy and directed biopsy are currently the major methods employed for diagnosing precancerous cervical lesions. However, several studies have demonstrated that even clinicians who are proficient in colposcopy have difficulties in making the correct diagnosis [18]. Therefore, the standardized and less fluctuating diagnostic performance of AI could play a role in this area. The feasibility of using deep learning-based colposcopy as an assistive diagnostic tool in high-grade CIN was evaluated in this study. The sensitivity of colposcopists in diagnosing CIN reportedly varies widely [19]. An inexperienced individual may miss high-grade lesions. Using the AI system, a non-professional gynecologist or general physician can make effective decisions regarding interventions (whether to perform a punch biopsy or transfer the patient to a specialized center).

The Cerviray® (AIDOT) system achieved a better sensitivity and comparable PPV in predicting high-grade lesions compared with the gold standard evaluation method for biopsy based on colposcopy. This level of diagnostic accuracy was comparable to that reported in a large cohort study [20]. As demonstrated previously, AI interpretation includes better AUC in differentiating high-risk and low-risk lesions than the human interpretations of colposcopic images by both clinicians. Consequently, these results suggest that deep learning-based AI interpretations may be utilized in clinical use. This is also supported by a recent study that evaluated deep learning models to automatically classify colposcopic images [21]. The authors concluded that an improved AUC was observed using a machine learning-based system in discriminating high-grade lesions from low-grade lesions; therefore, AI systems may be suited for automated evaluations of colposcopic images. In another observational study, automated visual evaluation of cervical images demonstrated greater AUC than the original interpretation of cervical images by human or conventional cytology [15].

The results of this study show that even skilled colposcopists showed markedly increased sensitivity with the assistance of AI. In this study, if the colposcopists accepted the more aggressive impressions of AI despite disagreements with it, the AUC increased from 0.755 to 0.799 and 0.713 to 0.769 for Doctors 1 and 2, respectively. The sensitivity was also higher after acceptance of aggressive AI impression, in contrast to relatively low specificity and PPV after acceptance. Usually, high sensitivity is related to high negative predictive value (NPV) rather than PPV. The screening tools usually favors the diagnostic method, which shows high sensitivity and NPV. The Cerviray AI® system was developed with the intention of utilizing the AI system in combination with human interpretation for screening high-grade cervical abnormality. Therefore, these subtle impairments of PPV might be acceptable.

Interestingly, as presented in Figure 3, the correlations between the two colposcopists were higher than any other correlations between the other modalities. AI interpretation and human colposcopic impressions demonstrated statistically significant correlations but a lower Pearson's R than that between the two doctors. This observation implies that the AI system interprets colposcopic images using logic that is different from that is used in human colposcopic evaluations. The conventional colposcopic evaluation includes a triad of mosaic, punctuation, and aceto-white epithelium, which could be present as a mixture in a majority of cases with severe lesions [22]. In contrast, the Cerviray AI® (AIDOT) system trains images under a subdivided network of serial processes (Figure 4). This process does not appear to follow the human colposcopy training but may include more delicate segmentation of abnormal lesions. Therefore, AI interpretations could be different from those of humans, but the logic for such interpretations remains unknown.

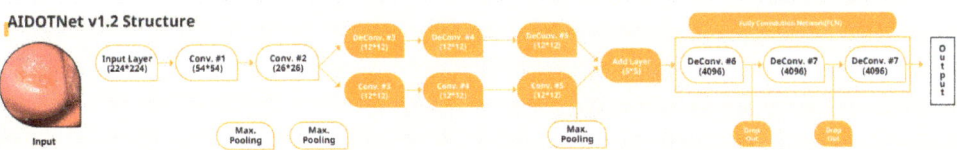

Figure 4. An algorithm of the deep learning process of Cerviray AI®. Briefly, it included the input of an image, multiple convolution and deconvolution networks of image processing while pooling and dropping out of data, and output of the result.

On the other hand, considering that the diagnostic value of AI interpretation was comparable to the impressions of colposcopic experts, AI interpretation might have a role as a diagnostic tool in evaluating high-grade cervical lesions in the distant future, especially in countries where certified or proficient colposcopists are insufficient. Generally, colposcopic evaluation includes a learning curve in achieving proficiency [23]. However, the AI system does not require this learning period, and this approach could improve the accessibility to cervical disease screening programs in developing countries or undeveloped countries. In the case of cytology and HPV testing, high lab equipment costs are incurred, and to operate the lab, it needs to build a lab and requires manpower, including pathologists, so there would be lots of operating costs. Therefore, it is recommended to use "visual Inspection with Acetic-acid" in underdeveloped areas, in which it is difficult to have cervical cancer screening [24,25]. Cerviray AI® does not need special maintenance or training cost to use. Even if there are no specialists for diagnosis, patients can get a diagnosis from doctors through a telemedicine system. Therefore, it is a very efficient and useful device, especially in underdeveloped or developing countries.

Only a few previous studies have reported the feasibility of machine learning applications in colposcopic classification for cervical lesions. The accuracy of the validation dataset has been reported to be approximately 50% in classifying CIN3, carcinoma in situ, and invasive cancer in 158 patients who underwent conization [26]. Although the study demonstrated the feasibility of the AI application, it did not provide satisfactory accuracy. In another investigation with 170 images, an accuracy of 72% was reported in classifying the colposcopic images [27]. However, the clinical significance of those results is limited because only 58 images were used for training the machine learning system. Recently, a large-scale study in 9406 women reported that better diagnostic accuracy was observed with an automated visual evaluation using a deep learning-based AI system compared with the human interpretations or conventional cytology [15]. Cho et al. also evaluated deep learning models in automatically classifying cervical neoplasms using colposcopic photographs [21]. AI demonstrated a superior AUC over human colposcopic impressions. These previous studies have limitations in that the colposcopic findings were retrospective data derived from multiple colposcopists with varying experiences. However, in this study, all images were reviewed separately by two experienced colposcopists for the purposes of this study. This approach provides important information about the validation of the accuracy of human colposcopic impressions. It also enables a direct comparison of AI interpretations with colposcopic findings.

However, this study has a few limitations. Firstly, patients with atypical glandular cells were excluded from the study population due to the possible association with endometrial disease [28]. Secondly, colposcopic images only provide visual information of the exocervix; therefore, patients with endocervical lesions are not considered good candidates for accurate AI interpretations. Inadequate colposcopic finding usually requires additional endocervical evaluations, including endocervical cytology or endocervical curettage. We should not overlook the limitation of colposcopy itself in terms of the possibility that the transformation zone could be multifocal and could be hardly assessed while lying in the isthmus of the uterus or in the fornix of the vagina. Thirdly, there was heterogeneity in the image quality or resolution between patients due to the retrospective nature of the study. Fourthly, the human colposcopic impressions in this study may not reflect the real-time colposcopic diagnoses. Two colposcopists in this study evaluated only the digitalized images retrospectively. Real-time colposcopic diagnosis is based on a combination of visualization of abnormal patterns and rate of acetowhite changes, subtle differences in the degree of acetowhite response, and even the degree of light reflection. Therefore, the sensitivity and specificity of two colposcopists in this study should not be considered as a conventional colposcopic evaluation. Prospective studies to compare real-time colposcopic impressions and concomitant AI interpretations are warranted to address this issue. Fifthly, the presented sensitivity of cytology in Table 3 is relatively low. However, this shows a sensitivity at cutoff cytological high-grade lesions, including ASC-H or HSIL, for detection of histological CIN2 or worse. This could be a reason why the sensitivity is low in this study. In a meta-analysis, the sensitivity of liquid-based cytology and conventional cytology for CIN2 or worse showed 57.1 and 55.2%, respectively [29]. Additionally, the study population is not balanced between groups. The study population of this study were mostly received colposcopic evaluation because of an abnormal cytologic result or positive HPV testing. The low percentage of individuals with normal cervix could alter the diagnostic value. Finally, the percentage of histological CIN2-3 in ASCUS and LSIL cytology results is relatively high. However, there also exist which shows similar findings with this study. It is reported that 17–36% of patients with ASCUS cytology were diagnosed to have CIN2-3 on biopsy, and 34–50% of patients with LSIL cytology had CIN2-3 on biopsy [30]. However, we could deny that the ratio of CIN2-3 from ASCUS and LSIL is relatively high in this study. This could be because of a high proportion of patients who are positive for high-risk HPV. This also shows the importance of the HPV test for cervical cancer screening. The study population had cytology for their cervical cancer screening. The updated recommendation of primary HPV testing for cervical cancer globally should be considered, and further study from individuals with regular HPV testing should be performed later.

5. Conclusions

In conclusion, our study highlights the feasibility of using machine learning-based AI systems in cervical cancer screening. AI interpretation of cervical images could be an assistive tool if it is used in combination with human colposcopic evaluation. Additionally, if additional supportive studies are followed, it might be utilized as an alternative tool in evaluating high-grade cervical lesions when proficient colposcopists are unavailable due to the lack of accessibility or high cost in low-income or developing countries. Much more data are warranted for using AI systems in the field of cervical cancer screening.

Author Contributions: Writing—original draft preparation, S.K.; writing—review and editing, S.K. and H.L.; conceptualization and visualization, S.L. and J.-Y.S.; supervision, intellectual content, and paper coordination, S.L., J.-Y.S., J.-K.L. and N.-W.L. All authors have read and agreed to the published version of the manuscript.

Funding: This study was funded by the Korea University Grant (R1928051).

Institutional Review Board Statement: The study was conducted according to the guidelines of the Declaration of Helsinki and approved by the Institutional Review Board (2019AN0019).

Informed Consent Statement: Not applicable.

Data Availability Statement: The data presented in this study are available on request from the corresponding author.

Conflicts of Interest: The authors declare no conflict of interest.

References

1. WHO Guidelines for Treatment of Cervical Intraepithelial Neoplasia 2–3 and Adenocarcinoma in Situ: Cryotherapy, Large Loop Excision of the Transformation Zone, and Cold Knife Conization; WHO Guidelines Approved by the Guidelines Review Committee; WHO: Geneva, Switzerland, 2014.
2. Chan, J.K.; Monk, B.J.; Brewer, C.; Keefe, K.A.; Osann, K.; McMeekin, S.; Rose, G.S.; Youssef, M.; Wilczynski, S.P.; Meyskens, F.L.; et al. HPV infection and number of lifetime sexual partners are strong predictors for 'natural' regression of CIN 2 and Br. *J. Cancer* **2003**, *89*, 1062–1066. [CrossRef] [PubMed]
3. Östör, A.G. Natural history of cervical intraepithelial neoplasia: A critical review. *Int. J. Gynecol. Pathol.* **1993**, *12*, 186–192. [CrossRef]
4. Silver, M.I.; Andrews, J.; Cooper, C.K.; Gage, J.C.; Gold, M.A.; Khan, M.J.; Massad, L.S.; Parvu, V.; Perkins, R.B.; Schiffman, M.; et al. Risk of Cervical Intraepithelial Neoplasia 2 or Worse by Cytology, Human Papillomavirus 16/18, and Colposcopy Impression. *Obstet. Gynecol.* **2018**, *132*, 725–735. [CrossRef]
5. Fontham, E.T.H.; Wolf, A.M.D.; Church, T.R.; Etzioni, R.; Flowers, C.R.; Herzig, A.; Guerra, C.E.; Oeffinger, K.C.; Shih, Y.T.; Walter, L.C.; et al. Cervical cancer screening for individuals at average risk: 2020 guideline update from the American Cancer Society. *CA Cancer J. Clin.* **2020**, *70*, 321–346. [CrossRef] [PubMed]
6. Goldie, S.J.; Gaffikin, L.; Goldhaber-Fiebert, J.D.; Gordillo-Tobar, A.; Levin, C.; Mahé, C.; Wright, T.C. Cost-Effectiveness of Cervical-Cancer Screening in Five Developing Countries. *N. Engl. J. Med.* **2005**, *353*, 2158–2168. [CrossRef] [PubMed]
7. Hull, R.; Mbele, M.; Makhafola, T.; Hicks, C.; Wang, S.; Reis, R.M.; Mehrotra, R.; Mkhize-Kwitshana, Z.; Kibiki, G.; Bates, D.O.; et al. Cervical cancer in low and middle-income countries (Review). *Oncol. Lett.* **2020**, *20*, 2058–2074. [CrossRef]
8. Gyawali, P.; Kc, S.; Ghimire, S. Role of Colposcopy in Detection of Dysplastic Cervical Lesion as a Screening Tool. *J. Glob. Oncol.* **2018**, *4*, 33s. [CrossRef]

9. Barut, M.U.; Kale, A.; Kuyumcuoğlu, U.; Bozkurt, M.; Ağaçayak, E.; Özekinci, S.; Gül, T. Analysis of Sensitivity, Specificity, and Positive and Negative Predictive Values of Smear and Colposcopy in Diagnosis of Premalignant and Malignant Cervical Lesions. *Med. Sci. Monit.* **2015**, *21*, 3860–3867. [CrossRef]
10. Karimi-Zarchi, M.; Zanbagh, L.; Shafii, A.; Shokouh, T.-Z.; Teimoori, S.; Yazdian-Anari, P. Comparison of Pap Smear and Colposcopy in Screening for Cervical Cancer in Patients with Secondary Immunodeficiency. *Electron. Physician* **2015**, *7*, 1542–1548. [CrossRef]
11. Stuebs, F.A.; Schulmeyer, C.E.; Mehlhorn, G.; Gass, P.; Kehl, S.; Renner, S.K.; Renner, S.P.; Geppert, C.; Adler, W.; Hartmann, A.; et al. Accuracy of colposcopy-directed biopsy in detecting early cervical neoplasia: A retrospective study. *Arch. Gynecol. Obstet.* **2018**, *299*, 525–532. [CrossRef]
12. Waring, J.; Lindvall, C.; Umeton, R. Automated machine learning: Review of the state-of-the-art and opportunities for healthcare. *Artif. Intell. Med.* **2020**, *104*, 101822. [CrossRef] [PubMed]
13. Zeng, X.; Luo, G. Progressive sampling-based Bayesian optimization for efficient and automatic machine learning model selection. *Health Inf. Sci. Syst.* **2017**, *5*, 2. [CrossRef] [PubMed]
14. Bao, H.; Bi, H.; Zhang, X.; Zhao, Y.; Dong, Y.; Luo, X.; Zhou, D.; You, Z.; Wu, Y.; Liu, Z.; et al. Artificial intelligence-assisted cytology for detection of cervical intraepithelial neoplasia or invasive cancer: A multicenter, clinical-based, observational study. *Gynecol. Oncol.* **2020**, *159*, 171–178. [CrossRef]
15. Hu, L.; Bell, D.; Antani, S.; Xue, Z.; Yu, K.; Horning, M.P.; Gachuhi, N.; Wilson, B.; Jaiswal, M.S.; Befano, B.; et al. An Observational Study of Deep Learning and Automated Evaluation of Cervical Images for Cancer Screening. *JNCI J. Natl. Cancer Inst.* **2019**, *111*, 923–932. [CrossRef] [PubMed]
16. Xue, P.; Tang, C.; Li, Q.; Li, Y.; Shen, Y.; Zhao, Y.; Chen, J.; Wu, J.; Li, L.; Wang, W.; et al. Development and validation of an artificial intelligence system for grading colposcopic impressions and guiding biopsies. *BMC Med.* **2020**, *18*, 406. [CrossRef] [PubMed]
17. Yuan, C.; Yao, Y.; Cheng, B.; Cheng, Y.; Li, Y.; Li, Y.; Liu, X.; Cheng, X.; Xie, X.; Wu, J.; et al. The application of deep learning based diagnostic system to cervical squamous intraepithelial lesions recognition in colposcopy images. *Sci. Rep.* **2020**, *10*, 11639. [CrossRef] [PubMed]
18. Fan, A.; Wang, C.; Zhang, L.; Yan, Y.; Han, C.; Xue, F. Diagnostic value of the 2011 International Federation for Cervical Pathology and Colposcopy Terminology in predicting cervical lesions. *Oncotarget* **2018**, *9*, 9166–9176. [CrossRef]
19. Mitchell, M.F. Colposcopy for the diagnosis of squamous intraepithelial lesions: A meta-analysis. *Obstet. Gynecol.* **1998**, *91*, 626–631. [CrossRef]
20. Benedet, J.L. An analysis of 84,244 patients from the British Columbia cytology–colposcopy program. *Gynecol. Oncol.* **2004**, *92*, 127–134. [CrossRef]
21. Cho, B.-J.; Choi, Y.J.; Lee, M.-J.; Kim, J.H.; Son, G.-H.; Park, S.-H.; Kim, H.-B.; Joo, Y.-J.; Cho, H.-Y.; Kyung, M.S.; et al. Classification of cervical neoplasms on colposcopic photography using deep learning. *Sci. Rep.* **2020**, *10*, 1–10. [CrossRef]
22. Kuramoto, H.; Jobo, T. Utility of Colposcopy: Comparison of Colposcopic Abnormality with Histology and Cytology, with Colposcopic Findings Focusing on the Lesion in Cervical Canal. In *Colposcopy and Cervical Pathology*; IntechOpen: London, UK, 2017. [CrossRef]
23. Khongthip, Y.; Manchana, T.; Oranratanaphan, S.; Lertkhachonsuke, R. Learning curve in colposcopic training among gynecologic oncology fellows. *Eur. J. Gynaecol. Oncol.* **2019**, *40*, 647–651.
24. Egede, J.; Ajah, L.; Ibekwe, P.; Agwu, U.; Nwizu, E.; Iyare, F. Comparison of the Accuracy of Papanicolaou Test Cytology, Visual Inspection with Acetic Acid, and Visual Inspection with Lugol Iodine in Screening for Cervical Neoplasia in Southeast Nigeria. *J. Glob. Oncol.* **2018**, *4*, 1–9. [CrossRef] [PubMed]
25. Vahedpoor, Z.; Behrashi, M.; Khamehchian, T.; Abedzadeh-Kalahroudi, M.; Moravveji, A.; Mohmadi-Kartalayi, M. Comparison of the diagnostic value of the visual inspection with acetic acid (VIA) and Pap smear in cervical cancer screening. *Taiwan J. Obstet. Gynecol.* **2019**, *58*, 345–348. [CrossRef] [PubMed]
26. Sato, M.; Horie, K.; Hara, A.; Miyamoto, Y.; Kurihara, K.; Tomio, K.; Yokota, H. Application of deep learning to the classification of images from colposcopy. *Oncol. Lett.* **2018**, *15*, 3518–3523. [CrossRef]
27. Simões, P.W.; Izumi, N.B.; Casagrande, R.S.; Venson, R.; Veronezi, C.D.; Moretti, G.P.; da Rocha, E.L.; Cechinel, C.; Ceretta, L.B.; Comunello, E.; et al. Classification of Images Acquired with Colposcopy Using Artificial Neural Networks. *Cancer Inform.* **2014**, *13*, S17948. [CrossRef] [PubMed]
28. Scheiden, R.; Wagener, C.; Knolle, U.; Dippel, W.; Capesius, C. Atypical glandular cells in conventional cervical smears: Incidence and follow-up. *BMC Cancer* **2004**, *4*, 1–9. [CrossRef]
29. Arbyn, M.; Bergeron, C.; Klinkhamer, P.; Martin-Hirsch, P.; Siebers, A.G.; Bulten, J. Liquid compared with conventional cervical cytology: A systematic review and meta-analysis. *Obstet. Gynecol.* **2008**, *111*, 167–177. [CrossRef]
30. Ovestad, I.T.; Vennestrøm, U.; Andersen, L.; Gudlaugsson, E.; Munk, A.C.; Malpica, A.; Feng, W.; Voorhorst, F.; Janssen, E.A.; Baak, J.P. Comparison of different commercial methods for HPV detection in follow-up cytology after ASCUS/LSIL, prediction of CIN2–3 in follow up biopsies and spontaneous regression of CIN2-3. *Gynecol. Oncol.* **2011**, *123*, 278–283. [CrossRef]

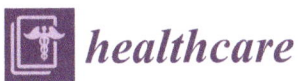

Article

Deep Learning on Histopathology Images for Breast Cancer Classification: A Bibliometric Analysis

Siti Shaliza Mohd Khairi [1,2], Mohd Aftar Abu Bakar [2,*], Mohd Almie Alias [2], Sakhinah Abu Bakar [2], Choong-Yeun Liong [2,†], Nurwahyuna Rosli [3] and Mohsen Farid [4]

[1] Faculty of Computer and Mathematical Sciences, Universiti Teknologi MARA, Shah Alam 40450, Malaysia; sitishaliza3425@uitm.edu.my
[2] Department of Mathematical Sciences, Faculty of Science & Technology, Universiti Kebangsaan Malaysia, Bangi 43600, Malaysia; mohdalmie@ukm.edu.my (M.A.A.); sakhinah@ukm.edu.my (S.A.B.); lg@ukm.edu.my (C.-Y.L.)
[3] Department of Pathology, Faculty of Medicine, Hospital Canselor Tuanku Muhriz, Universiti Kebangsaan Malaysia, Jalan Yaacob Latif, Bandar Tun Razak, Cheras, Kuala Lumpur 56000, Malaysia; nurwahyuna@ukm.edu.my
[4] Department of Computing and Mathematics, University of Derby, Kedleston Road, Derby DE22 1GB, UK; m.farid@derby.ac.uk
* Correspondence: aftar@ukm.edu.my
† The author is deceased.

Citation: Khairi, S.S.M.; Bakar, M.A.A.; Alias, M.A.; Bakar, S.A.; Liong, C.-Y.; Rosli, N.; Farid, M. Deep Learning on Histopathology Images for Breast Cancer Classification: A Bibliometric Analysis. *Healthcare* 2022, 10, 10. https://doi.org/10.3390/healthcare10010010

Academic Editor: Daniele Giansanti

Received: 15 November 2021
Accepted: 12 December 2021
Published: 22 December 2021

Publisher's Note: MDPI stays neutral with regard to jurisdictional claims in published maps and institutional affiliations.

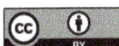

Copyright: © 2021 by the authors. Licensee MDPI, Basel, Switzerland. This article is an open access article distributed under the terms and conditions of the Creative Commons Attribution (CC BY) license (https://creativecommons.org/licenses/by/4.0/).

Abstract: Medical imaging is gaining significant attention in healthcare, including breast cancer. Breast cancer is the most common cancer-related death among women worldwide. Currently, histopathology image analysis is the clinical gold standard in cancer diagnosis. However, the manual process of microscopic examination involves laborious work and can be misleading due to human error. Therefore, this study explored the research status and development trends of deep learning on breast cancer image classification using bibliometric analysis. Relevant works of literature were obtained from the Scopus database between 2014 and 2021. The VOSviewer and Bibliometrix tools were used for analysis through various visualization forms. This study is concerned with the annual publication trends, co-authorship networks among countries, authors, and scientific journals. The co-occurrence network of the authors' keywords was analyzed for potential future directions of the field. Authors started to contribute to publications in 2016, and the research domain has maintained its growth rate since. The United States and China have strong research collaboration strengths. Only a few studies use bibliometric analysis in this research area. This study provides a recent review on this fast-growing field to highlight status and trends using scientific visualization. It is hoped that the findings will assist researchers in identifying and exploring the potential emerging areas in the related field.

Keywords: breast cancer; bibliometric analysis; healthcare; medical imaging; VOSviewer

1. Introduction

Cancer may arise from almost any part of the human body where cells start to grow uncontrollably [1]. Deaths caused by cancers keep increasing every year and are considered as the main illness globally [2–4]. Breast cancer is one of the top illnesses contributing to the highest death rates among women, especially in developing countries such as Melanesia, Western Africa, Australia, Micronesia/Polynesia, and the Caribbean [5]. However, it is noticeable that the percentage of breast cancer cases in Australia, Western Europe, Northern America, and Northern Europe are the highest [5,6]. Women are commonly diagnosed with breast cancer, but men, however, are not excluded [7]. The breast structure of women is mainly made up of milk ducts, lobules, and adipose tissue [8]. Breast cancer may initiate in the ducts which carry milk to the nipple or in the lobules glands, the part of the breast that produces breast milk [8,9]. Globally, the majority of breast cancers are of ductal and lobular subtypes, given that 40–75% are comprised of ductal subtypes of all reported cases [10].

Early diagnosis and treatment may benefit in preventing breast cancer from developing to the advanced cancer level. There are several medical imaging procedures for breast cancers such as mammograms (X-rays), ultrasound (sound waves/sonography), magnetic resonance imaging (MRI), and biopsy [11–14]. However, the use of breast cancer images to confirm the cancer region is only available through biopsy procedures [15]. Tissue biopsy examination is currently the clinical gold standard in cancer diagnosis. Tissue biopsy produces histopathology images that can enhance the results of breast cancer classification [16]. The basic procedure in biopsy is collecting a tissue sample from the body for further analysis by the histopathologist [17]. The tissue will be immersed in the formalin solution and planted in paraffin wax before being cut carefully, resulting in histopathology slides which then converted to images [18,19]. However, the manual procedure of biopsy analysis is tedious, time-consuming, and restricted by the quality of the histopathology image and the histopathologists' skill [20,21]. The histopathology images are stored and analyzed using the Computer-Aided Diagnosis (CAD) system [22]. The CAD system is used to overcome the issue of classification accurateness from manual approaches [23], and machine learning techniques are required [24].

The involvement of machine learning algorithms could help to reduce the number of unnecessary biopsy images. For an image analysis, there are four important stages to be considered: (i) input, (ii) feature extraction and selection, (iii) classifier model, and (iv) classifier output. According to Nahid and Kong [8], feature extraction and representation approaches are important to produce accurate and reliable results. There are two types of features which are hand-crafted features and learned features. Expert-level knowledge is required for hand-crafted feature extraction during image analysis [25]. A predefined hand-crafted feature is important in traditional machine learning methods, such as support vector machine (SVM), Naïve Bayes, random forest (RF), and k-means clustering. For example, [26] used regional and localized features with SVM as a classifier to evaluate the quality of 3D images. On the other hand, wavelet transform was applied to tree-structured algorithm for automatic image grading in two datasets with different magnification factors [27]. The authors used k-means clustering and texture features to locate the affected regions in the segmentation process. Similarly, [28] also used the wavelet transform to extract the features from breast cancer images and SVM classifier meant for feature selection. The result indicates that the combination of SVM classifier and chain-like agent genetic algorithm (CAGA) to obtain the optimal feature set was remarkable, with an accuracy of 96.19%.

The majority of the studies are limited to a macroscopic overview of breast cancer image classification. Specific visual bibliometric analysis is relatively low. Based on the bibliometric analysis, this research aims to present updated and microscopic overview characteristics of breast cancer image classification publications. The clear and informative maps offered in this work highlight research accomplishments in the deep learning on breast cancer image classification domain, which may aid researchers and practitioners in identifying the underlying implications of authors, journals, countries, references, and research themes. The co-authorship network analysis is believed to give some insight on the intellectual collaboration and interaction between researchers. In detail, the focuses of the paper are: (i) to examine the number of papers on the rise of publications and citations on deep learning approaches published from the years 2014 to 2021, (ii) to map the co-authorship networks among countries, authors, and scientific journals, and (iii) to analyze the co-occurrence network of the authors' keywords globally.

This paper hopes that the findings will help to initiate ideas for future research in the related field and, in turn, will benefit the patients and healthcare providers. This study is also important as guidance for researchers that are unfamiliar with deep learning but interested in its potential in breast cancer image classification, where most active researchers and recent significant research topics among authors are discovered. This study specifically highlighted the application of deep learning instead of machine learning since recently, the field has been more strongly associated with image classification. Based on the overview of the progress, it is estimated that deep learning will continue to evolve and flourish as a significant tool for image classification.

2. Breast Cancer Image Classification

2.1. Bibliometric Analysis of Breast Cancer Studies

Bibliometrics can visualize the structure of the scientific disciplines based on the bibliographic information gained from the databases [29]. Bibliometrics have been used in vast scientific areas to analyze prior studies' trends and patterns, such as web accessibility, text mining, sustainable business, and healthcare [29–32]. Some bibliometric studies have discussed breast-cancer-related topics. Cinar [33] provided a bibliometric analysis on 2734 articles related to breast cancer focused on the nursing field from the year 2009–2018. Based on the keyword analysis, the term "breast cancer survivor" was highly cited in year 2014 to 2018, and research showed a progressive trend of breast cancer related to the nursing field within those five years. Salod and Singh [34] studied the publication trends, country collaboration, author productivity, institutional collaboration, and productive journal based on the literatures related to breast cancer in the field of machine learning.

In a recent review, Joshi et al. [35] studied machine learning methods towards breast cancer histopathology images. Machine learning is a subset of artificial intelligence which includes statistical methods that can improve and learn the information directly from data. They pointed out that there was a growing interest in machine learning and histopathology images of breast cancer. Based on keyword analysis, their study revealed that disease in female, breast cancer, deep learning, histopathology and medical imaging are the top important keywords [35]. This showed that machine learning applications offered a potential research trend towards medical images analysis. However, the final performance of image analysis relies on the pre-processing data, including hand-crafted features extraction which is hard to solve by using traditional machine learning methods [25,36]. With the technological evolution of deep learning and rapid growth research of the application in healthcare, especially breast cancer, understanding the development of deep learning has become essential.

2.2. Breast Cancer Image Database

Breast cancer is a common cancer type among people, especially women, around the world. An early detection of breast cancer would lead to an appropriate treatment which might increase the survival rate of affected people [35]. Hence, a well-defined database is important to measure the performance of breast cancer classification models. There are several databases that are publicly available for breast cancer diagnosis such as Mammography Image Analysis Society (MIAS), Wisconsin Breast Cancer Dataset (WBCD), Digital Database for Screening Mammography (DDSM), Breast Cancer Histopathology (BreakHis), and Breast Cancer Histology (BACH). Since deep learning is gaining the fame for its ability to process image data in hierarchical representation using nonlinear transformations [25,37], hence the histopathology images are broadly used by researchers. The BreakHis and BACH datasets were made up of histopathology images. According to Li et al. [38], BreakHis dataset is extensively used in CNN algorithms related to image classification. They propose a new CNN architecture that uses local information in the breast cancer images and extra features extraction through different dense blocks and SENet module.

The BreakHis dataset was first introduced in 2016, which comprised 7909 histopathology images collected from the P & D Laboratory, Brazil [39]. Nahid and Kong stated that after the introduction of BreakHis dataset, there were about 20 articles published within a year from 2016 to 2017. Out of the total images, 2480 were benign images and 5429 malignant images with four different magnification factors. Table 1 showed detailed image distribution based on the magnification factors $40\times$, $100\times$, $200\times$, and $400\times$. Similarly, the

BACH dataset [40] is also available in three-channel RGB color of histopathology images. The biopsy tissues collected were stained with standard staining protocol, hematoxylin and eosin (H&E), which results in a total of 400 histopathology images.

Table 1. Summary of image distribution for different magnification factors.

Magnification	40×	100×	200×	400×
Benign	652	644	623	588
Malignant	1370	1437	1390	1232

2.3. Breast Cancer Image Classification using Deep Learning Approaches

In earlier studies, the classification of breast cancer images centralized on traditional machine learning methods such as Support Vector Machine (SVM) [41–43], Naïve Bayes [44–46], and Random Forest [47,48]. Machine learning involves the algorithms design and deployment to assess data and corresponding attributes without any prior task based on predetermined inputs from the environment [49]. Traditional machine learning methods rely on the quality of feature extraction that is limited to certain problems resulting from its shallow classifier [25]. Lately, the deep learning methods have been proven for more promising results specifically on large and complex data [50]. The implementation of feature learning methods (transfer learning) in deep learning helps to reduce the computational time, yet it obtained significant accuracy value compared to machine learning with hand-crafted features [51]. Generally, deep learning in CAD system outperformed the traditional approach because the automatic learning feature was created to analyze the variation and complexity of images directly; hence, convolutional neural network (CNN) is the most common model used for breast cancer diagnosis [52,53]. In 2020, Lin and Jeng [54] proposed a CNN model with uniform experimental design (UED) to classify breast cancer histopathology images. Their model outperformed other established deep learning models with lowest computational time. Current computing power can help to solve the related problems and further improve the quality of health and life among the community.

Deep learning is an established and emerging approach among researchers in the field of machine learning [55,56]. The main objective when employing deep learning is to discover multiple levels representations based on learning algorithm which are aimed for higher-level features for image classification and identification [50,57,58]. Generally, it is focused on learning algorithm that is able to learn, develop, and improve on its own to process data. Deep learning algorithms can extract features from high-dimensional images for internal representation [16]. Traditional machine learning works well with structured data with up to hundreds of features or characteristics. Unfortunately, for unstructured data, the analysis process will become tedious, or worse: unfeasible. Unstructured data are data stored in unstructured format and not prescribed by data models such as image, media, text data, and audio. Deep learning models different fundamental or needed qualities in data using a model architecture that is made up of different processing layers and non-linear variations [50,55,59].

It has been observed that researchers' attention has recently shifted to deep learning because of its great success in solving problems related to unstructured data. Convolutional Neural Network (CNN) is a part of deep learning models that can be used for image classification and feature extraction effectively [60]. In the medical field, deep learning provides a useful approach for assisting radiologists in making an early breast cancer diagnosis with histopathology images [59,61]. Breast cancer classification, signal processing [62], and image analysis [63] have benefited from deep learning methods in recent years.

In 2021, Zuluaga-Gomez et al. [60] designed a deep learning architecture from CNN to detect patterns visually on thermal images (DMR-IR database). They proposed a Bayesian optimization, Tree Parzen Estimator (TPE), as the hyper-parameter to optimize the algorithm. Experimental results showed competitive improvement of the CNN approach with an accuracy of 92%. The study also proved that data pre-processing and data augmentation help in improving the model performance. Similarly, Alom et al. [63] presented a novel CNN approach based on inception and residual networks for breast cancer multi-classification with different data augmentation methods. The experiments showed improvement of accuracy by approximately 1.05% (image-level) and 0.55% (patient-level) as compared with models that were based on learning and were data-driven for multi-classification.

With the aim of detecting and identifying breast cancer, Hirra et al. [59] applied a patch-based deep learning approach, Deep Belief Network (DBN), for automatic features extraction on histopathology images. The proposed model, namely, Ps-DBN-BC, gained a promising result with an accuracy greater than 85%, hence outperforming the 17-layer CNN architecture. This work indicated that architecture with deeper layers does not necessarily provide outstanding performance. Hameed et al. [61] developed an ensemble deep learning approach for histopathology images to classify carcinoma or non-carcinoma images automatically. They used two pre-trained deep CNN-based models for excellent convergence results in a small dataset, and the accuracy obtained was 95.29%. On the other hand, deep learning also benefited the signal processing area, as presented by Pavithra et al. on the effectiveness of thermography for breast cancer detection with appropriate choice of feature extraction, segmentation, and classification algorithms [62].

3. Materials and Methods

3.1. Bibliometric Analysis

The implementation of bibliometric analysis at the beginning of the research process is popular among researchers because it helps to discover the information underlying the published articles in specific areas or topics [64,65]. Although there are different methods to explore and organize earlier findings from the literature search, bibliometrics has advantages in terms of being a systematic, understandable, and reproducible review process [66]. A detailed bibliometric analysis can capture the growth of particular research studies in a given time period [67]. The bibliometric networks were visualized using R Programming Language [68] and VOSviewer software [69]. This study executed co-authorship and co-occurrence analyses for network mapping. A bibliometric analysis was used to study the relationship of scientific publications among countries and authors by constructing and visualizing the network maps.

3.2. Data Collection

The data retrieval process involved the Scopus database, retrieved on 22 October 2021. Scopus is one of the largest relevant academic abstracts and indexing databases from Elsevier [30,70]. Scopus is also more effective for health-related topic searches compared to other databases such as PubMed and Web of Science [71,72]. The bibliometric analysis reviewed all related published articles between the year 2014 to 2021.

Articles included in the research focused on histopathology breast cancer images. For further analysis, articles that mentioned deep learning, convolutional neural network, transfer learning, breast cancer, breast neoplasm, breast tumor and breast diagnostic were included. The articles were selected based on the abstract reviewed. All articles are available for download, and non-English articles were excluded.

The study is focused on deep learning algorithms for breast cancer image classification. Hence, articles that use conventional neural networks or other machine learning techniques such as regression, clustering, and decision trees were excluded from this research. Deep learning algorithms have gained huge interest in biomedical image analysis [73,74]. In fact, deep learning algorithms have shown to be a better alternative for medical image classification and detection. There are several characteristics of deep learning such as incorporating a large amount of data, the depth of the network, and optimizing hyper-parameters. In addition, the study population involving other image types, for instance, mammogram, ultrasound, and thermogram, were discarded from the analysis. A total of 498 articles were extracted from the Scopus database. After the filtration process on inclusion and exclusion criteria, 488 articles were selected for elements extraction of the articles. After a thorough screening process based on the abstract, 373 articles were finally included for further analysis. Figure 1 shows the flow diagram of the research process.

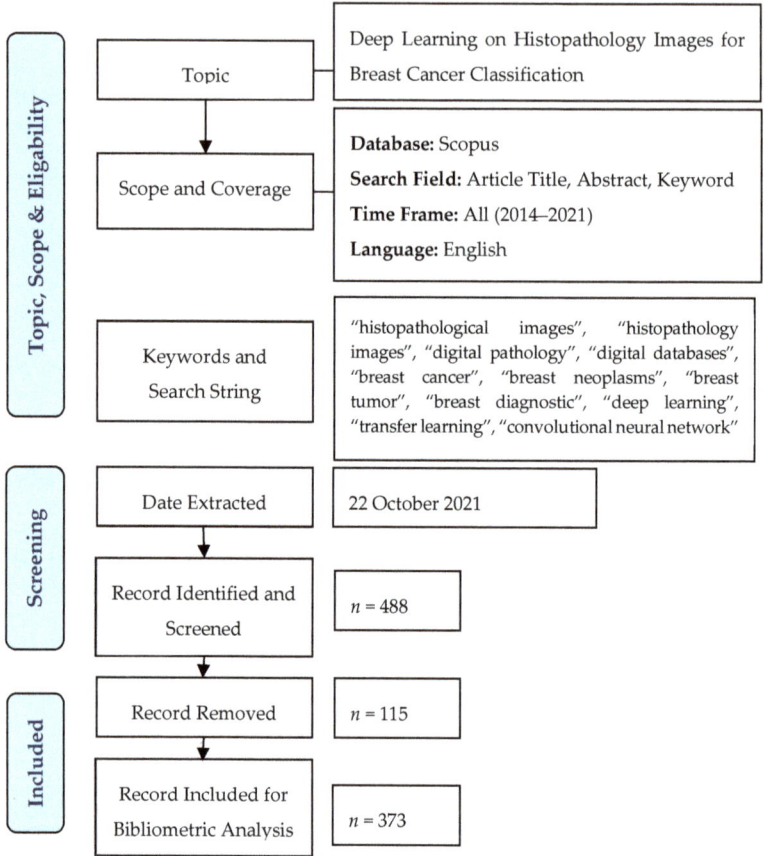

Figure 1. Flow diagram of the research process.

4. Results and Discussion

4.1. Overview on Document and Source Type

Firstly, the data were tabulated based on the document type, where document type is referred to as a structured document with several valid elements and originality such as article, conference paper, review, and a book chapter. Meanwhile, source type is the source information for the documents, including journals, conference proceedings, and book series. There is a possibility of the abstracts from conference proceedings published twice as in the conference abstract and full journal [75]. Given the fast development in computer science and studies in the deep learning area, proceeding publications were also considered in this bibliometric analysis. Recent studies also showed that proceeding publications do have a significant impact on highly cited publications, especially in terms of citation counts [76,77]. The majority of the publications are scientific articles (48.53%), followed by conference papers (41.55%), conference reviews (4.02%), reviews (3.22%), and book chapters (1.87%) as shown in Table 2. Other document types represent less than 1% of the total publication.

Table 2. Document type from Journal.

Document Type	Frequency	Percentage ($n = 373$)
Article	181	48.53
Conference paper	155	41.55
Conference review	15	4.02
Book chapter	7	1.87
Erratum	1	0.27
Note	1	0.27
Review	12	3.22
Short Survey	1	0.27
Total	373	100.00

4.2. Publication Growth

The pattern of publication growth is measured based on the published documents in the particular year. Figure 2 represents the publication trends and total mean citations of articles annually from 2014 to 2021. Scopus recorded Wang et al. [51] as the first published document on deep learning for breast cancer towards histopathology images in 2014, and to date, the document has more than 250 citations. Inspired by the rapid development of systems for invasive breast cancer detection, the authors combined a deep learning approach with hand-crafted features to maximize the model performance yet reduced the computational complexity since only light CNN method were implemented. They utilized 326 mitotic nuclei of breast cancer images in three-layer CNN architectures (two pooling layers and a fully connected layer). Since the number of images were low, they also used Synthetic Minority Oversampling Technique (SMOTE) to reduce the biasness during classification. Based on the comparison of several CNN-based methods, the results indicated that false positive (FP) errors were reduced, which showed that CNN was able to classify the images accurately. In 2016, one of the authors, Madabhushi A., collaborated with Janowczyk A. in [78] to analyze the digital pathology images using deep learning methods through segmentation and detection tasks of breast cancer images. They concluded that deep learning can be a reliable method because of the advantage in terms of feature extraction which can be directly extracted from the images. The study also has been cited by 747 documents since the first publication to date. This showed that more researchers are interested in deep learning-related research. Apart from that, Figure 2 also depicted the number of publications that increased steadily between 2015 and 2021, with the peak publications being in 2021, with 118 documents. This indicates the advancements in computing power and imaging technologies lead the researchers to explore the potential of deep learning to provide more promising results for histopathological image analysis [79–81]. From a citation perspective, the mean total citations of the documents were highest in 2014 and followed by year 2016; meanwhile, the lowest was for those published in 2021. This is not surprising as the citable years are not long enough after the publication [82].

4.3. Country Network Analysis

The co-authorship network of countries on breast cancer image classification using deep learning resulted in 71 countries from 2014–2021. Table 3 tabulates the top five countries according to their total link strength. The United States is considered a prominent country in scientific publications compared to others. The result is in line with other bibliometric analyses on "breast cancer" [33]. This could be contributed by greater financial support for researchers in the United States and the large population in the United States [83].

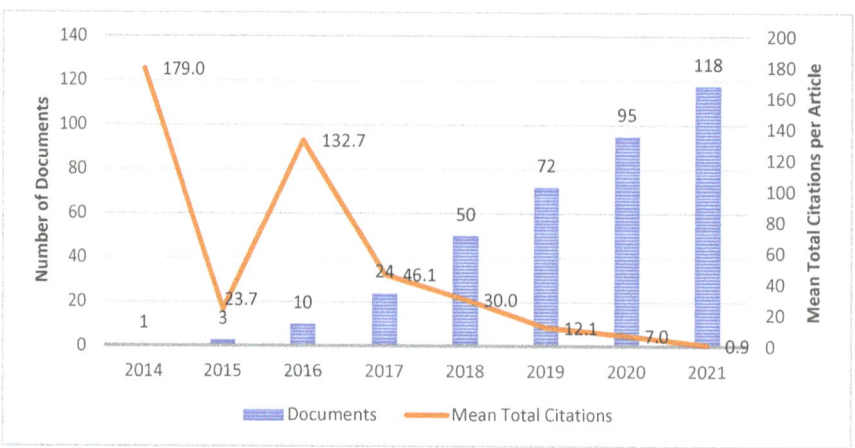

Figure 2. Flow diagram of the research process.

Table 3. Document type from journal.

Country	TLS [1]	Links	Documents	Citations	Cluster
United States	51	21	68	2235	6
China	39	17	71	1586	9
India	26	16	80	674	1
South Korea	17	11	12	444	3
United Kingdom	17	10	20	190	2
Germany	14	10	14	239	3
Sweden	14	9	10	192	5
Pakistan	13	6	13	172	7
Portugal	12	10	5	157	3
Australia	10	7	13	201	2

[1] Total link strength.

Based on a threshold of three publications per country, 35 countries were matched as shown in Figure 3. The size of circle represents the total link strength and lines among the countries, representing the collaboration link between countries. In country network analysis, there are nine different colors which indicate a total of nine clusters formed (distinguished by the colors of red, green, blue, yellow, purple, aqua, orange, brown, and pink). For bibliometric analysis, normally each research constituent (countries, authors, and journals) was clustered using a combination of multidimensional scaling (MDS) and hierarchical clustering (see [84]). In this study, the clustering methods were based on a unified approach proposed by [85] with modularity-based clustering to explore the structure of the network such as social interaction among authors and their countries. For example, Cluster 6 (Aqua) has strong collaboration with other countries such as countries from Cluster 2 (Green) and Cluster 3 (Blue). All countries were connected to each other in the network map.

It is interesting to note that India is one of the countries with a high number of publications; however, the number of citations is far less than the United States and China. This could be explained by the passion of researchers to conduct studies on the topic within the country but the lack of collaboration with other countries. The overlay visualization in Figure 4 focuses on the country collaboration of India. There are total of 16 countries collaborated with India included Iraq, Norway, Saudi Arabia, South Korea, and France. By referring to the line that connected between each country to India, most of the countries started collaborated with India in early 2020. Deep learning methods have achieved great success in breast cancer image classification among researchers in India [86–89]. This also explains why the number of documents published in India is high but received lower citations, since the timeline between publication year and citable year is not long.

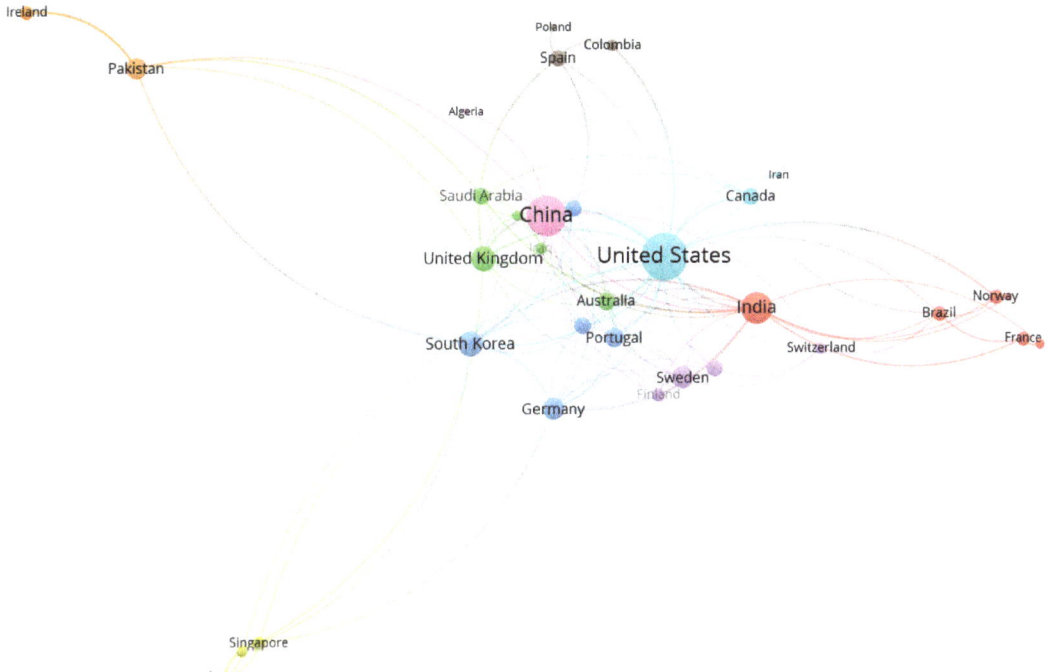

Figure 3. Co-authorship network visualization of countries in publication for 2014–2021.

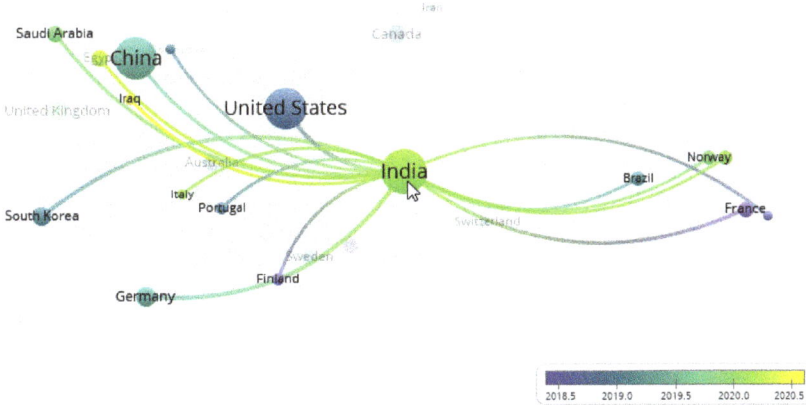

Figure 4. Co-authorship overlay visualization of India.

4.4. Author Network Analysis

A total of 1310 authors published on the topic related to breast cancer image classification using deep learning. Among them, 9 authors (0.69%) published at least five documents, 39 authors (2.98%) contributed between three to four publications, and 1262 authors (96.34%) published at most two documents. From Figure 5a, the lines connected between authors shows their cooperation link. For example, a reasonable research link was indicated from close and strong interconnections between the collaboration of Zhang Y., Li X., and Wang X. from Cluster 1 (Red), Wang L. in Cluster 5 (Purple), and Li Z. in Cluster 8 (Brown). The authors Madabhushi, Gilmore, and Zhang S. in Cluster 6 (Aqua) were from the United States, while most authors from Cluster 1 (Red) represented authors from China. This indicated that authors from similar countries are closely linked and more likely to work together. Based on the density visualization (Figure 5b), Madabhushi A., Gilmore H., Li Y., Wang J., Li X., and Zhang Y. led the collaboration in breast cancer histopathology image research.

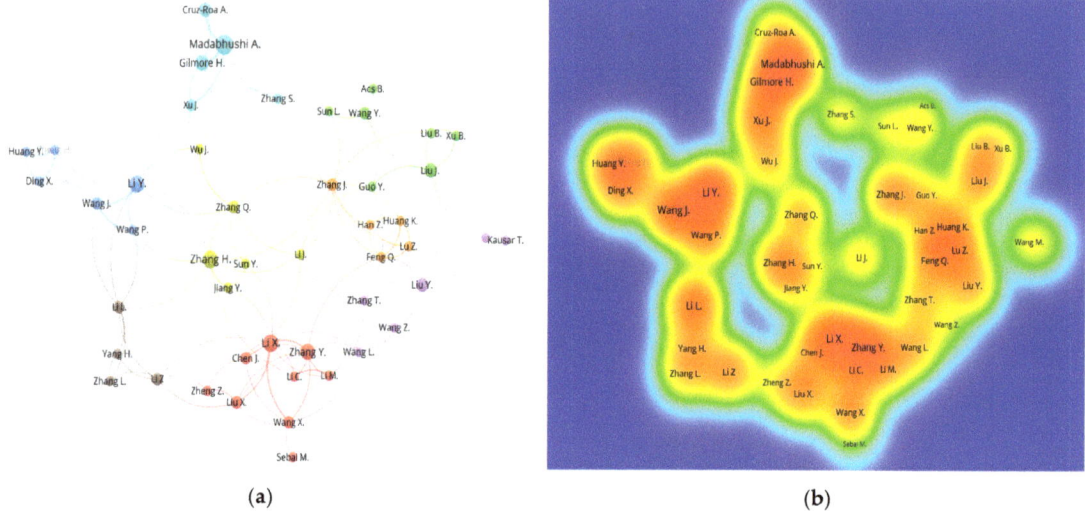

Figure 5. (**a**) Co-authorship network visualization of authors in publication for 2014–2021. (**b**) Density visualization of authors in publication for 2014–2021.

Table 4 presents the top 10 most productive authors ranked by the total link strength. It is interesting to note that the authors started to work collaboratively and contributed to publications after 2017; hence, the research domain has maintained its growth rate since. The total link strength of authors showed the collaboration closeness among them, which means higher total link strength indicated that more commonly collaboration occurs for the authors. An author from China, Li Y., had the most active collaboration with other authors such as Li L., Zhang H., Xu J., and Wang P., but the result showed that Madabhushi A. was the most highly cited author on the research topic. Some authors such as Xu J. and Gilmore H. had lower total link strength but recorded highly cited publications. This could be explained by referring to their popular publication related to nuclei detection using breast cancer histopathology images that has more than 600 paper citations [90].

Table 5 shows extra information on the research institutes and their research focus ranked based on the number of documents published in 2014–2021. The Case Western Reserve University has the highest number of publications that focuses on the convolutional neural network, digital pathology, image classification. Madabhushi A. from Case Western University has collaborated with authors from various institutes in all the nine documents published; hence, it is not surprising that Madabhushi A. has the highest paper citations.

Out of 10 research institutes, four of them are in China while two in Canada and one each are in the United States, India, the Netherlands, and Sweden. This finding implies that convolutional neural network and deep learning-related research has improved in China over these years [91].

Table 4. Document type from journal.

Author	TLS [1]	Links	Documents	Citations	Affiliation	APY [2]
Li Y.	18	10	7	93	Chongqing University, China	2018
Madabhushi A.	15	5	9	912	Case Western Reserve University, United States	2017
Li X.	15	10	7	56	Chongqing University of Posts and Telecommunications, China	2020
Wang J.	14	8	4	31	Chongqing University, China	2020
Gilmore H.	13	5	6	891	Case Western Reserve University, United States	2017
Zhang Y.	13	8	6	38	Nanjing University, China	2019
Li. L	13	7	4	36	Chongqing University, China	2020
Xu J.	11	7	4	485	Nanjing University, China	2018
Zhang H.	10	9	7	130	East China Jiaotong University, China	2019
Li Z.	10	6	4	22	Chongqing University of Posts and Telecommunications, China	2020

[1] Total link strength; [2] average publication year.

Table 5. Research institutes and their research focus.

Affiliation	Research Focus	Document
Case Western Reserve University	Convolutional neural network, digital pathology, image classification	9
Indian Institute of Technology Kharagpur	Features, convolutional neural network, whole slide images	7
Shenzhen University	Image classification, convolutional neural network	6
Radboud University Medical Center	Deep learning, whole slide images	6
University of Toronto	Convolutional neural network, review analysis	6
Karolinska Institute	Convolutional neural network, classification, deep learning	5
Xiamen University	Segmentation, detection, convolutional neural network	5
Sunnybrook Health University	Deep learning-based, convolutional neural network, feature extraction	5
Southern Medical University	Deep learning, cancer staging, classification	4
Chongqing University	Features, convolutional neural network, image classification	3

4.5. Journal Network Analysis

In journal network analysis, the number of articles published and the number of citations were considered while examining the most prominent journals in the topic of deep learning and breast cancer image classification. The citation analysis of journals resulted in 190 journals for 373 documents. Table 6 gives the top 20 journals published on breast cancer image classification using deep learning. Most publications in the related topic were published in Lecture Notes in Computer Science, Proceedings—International Symposium on Biomedical Imaging, IEEE Access, Scientific Reports and Communications in Computer and Information Science. Based on other indicators, IEEE Transactions on Medical Imaging and Scientific Reports have a significantly higher number of citations, with 703 and 451 citations, respectively. As shown in Figure 6, different node size represents different amounts of publications in the journal. Using a threshold of at least three articles per journal, only 24 journals were mapped in the network.

Table 6. Top 5 journals in publication for 2014–2021.

Journal	TLS [1]	Links	Documents	Cit [2]
IEEE Access	26	10	10	48
IEEE Transactions on Medical Imaging	24	13	5	703
Scientific Reports	21	16	10	451
Computerized Medical Imaging and Graphics	14	9	4	114
Medical Image Analysis	14	10	5	177
Biocybernetics and Biomedical Engineering	12	8	5	41
Lecture Notes in Computer Science (including subseries lecture notes in artificial intelligence and lecture notes in bioinformatics)	12	8	36	433
Expert Systems with Applications	11	8	3	117
International Journal of Advanced Computer Science and Applications	11	7	4	66
Frontiers in Genetics	10	6	3	71
Biomedical Signal Processing and Control	9	6	5	25
International Journal of Imaging Systems and Technology	9	5	6	27
Journal of Medical Imaging	8	6	3	249
Communications in Computer and Information Science	7	4	10	10
Advances in Intelligent Systems and Computing	6	5	8	16
IEEE Journal of Biomedical and Health Informatics	6	4	6	101
Proceedings of the International Joint Conference on Neural Networks	6	5	4	417
Proceedings—International Symposium on Biomedical Imaging	4	3	13	262
Lecture Notes in Electrical Engineering	3	2	3	0
Cancers	1	1	6	9

[1] Total link strength; [2] citations.

Research collaboration aims to combine various types of expertise for research output development by linking the knowledge and skills together. Co-authorship networks are commonly used to examine the collaboration patterns and discover the influential authors and organizations [92]. The analysis illustrates the social network structure that exists between individuals or organizations. Recently, the technological breakthrough in the CAD system has helped to improve the computational time of diagnosis and minimize the rate of misdiagnosis during image classification [93,94].

In the analysis, the involvement of the United States, China, and India as the most central countries in the network showed their scientific contribution to breast cancer and deep learning issues globally. The distance between each circle (node) implies the collaboration strength such that the further distance represents less collaboration between countries. Currently, the United States and China have contributed more than 40% of the total publications, and the collaboration strength between these countries is high. According to [34], a high number of publications in both countries are related to the investment of the business sectors in their Research and Development (R&D) expenditure. Apart from that, there is a growing trend of developing countries to engage in research related to the issues. For example, significant performance from China, India, and Pakistan is in line with previous studies that revealed breast cancer is among the important illness and research areas [95–97]. Both the developed and developing countries are publishing their research since breast cancer is a global burden issue [98].

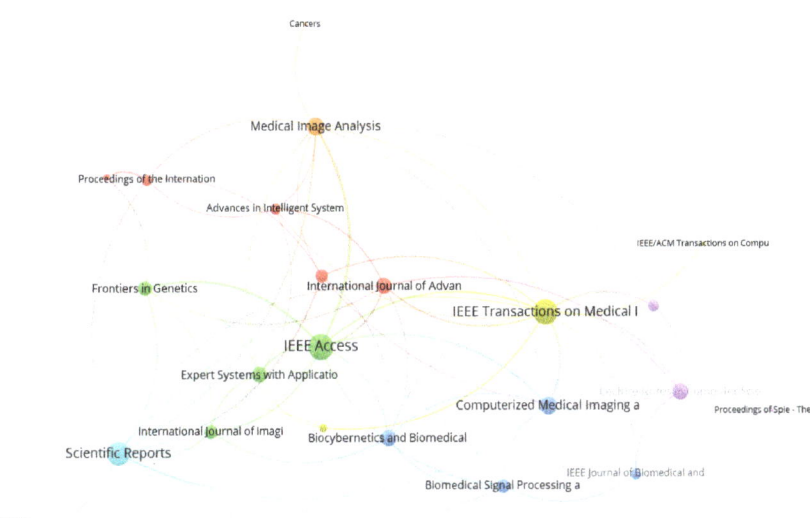

Figure 6. Citation network visualization of journals in publication for 2014–2021.

Based on the density visualization, Madabhushi A. and Gilmore H. again are the most productive authors and most linked on the research topic. Many authors from various affiliations and countries collaborate with them such as Cruz-Roa A. from Universidad de los Llanos, Columbia [99] and Xu J. from Nanjing University of Information Science and Technology, China [100,101].

4.6. Co-Occurrence Analysis of Author Keywords

For the years 2014 to 2021, a co-occurrence analysis of author keywords was conducted with a minimum of three keyword occurrences as a threshold for the study. Out of 657 keywords, 42 were found to be relevant. There are seven distinct clusters in the results (Figure 7). When two keywords appear together in one article or more, they are more likely to form a cluster. In Figure 7, the co-occurrence network map of keywords is depicted, given that the larger size of the circle, the higher the co-occurrence of keywords. Furthermore, having closer keywords together shows a stronger relationship. The average year of publication of the keywords was determined using colors. Notably, the focus of research from 2018 to 2019 was on biopsy image aspects (Dark blue) such as "histopathology image analysis", "digital pathology", "convolutional neural networks", "whole slide images", and "computer-aided diagnostics". Instead, the network map reveals a greater focus on breast cancer classification approaches such as "deep learning", "transfer learning", "CNN", "image classification", "medical image processing", and "feature extraction" from 2019 to date.

The top keywords that are identified through co-occurrence analysis is breast cancer and deep learning with 152 and 139 total number of counts, respectively. The result is as expected since breast cancer and deep learning are part of the search keywords for bibliometric analysis. Breast cancer studies received high attention in research related to deep learning. According to Samb et al. [102], chronic illness will lead to 80% human deaths by 2023, which also contributes to global issues, and proper treatments that are aimed at combating the illness may benefit the healthcare system. Specifically, breast cancer is also one of the current leading cause of deaths where the mortality rate is still high, even though the mortality trend has been reduced since 1989 [3]. Hence, researchers focus their work on early detection of breast cancer through deep learning technology [103,104]. This is supported by the overlay visualization in Figure 7, where the research direction aimed at the efficiency of CNN towards image analysis from 2018 to 2020. In 2018, Cruz-Roa et al. [99] proposed a new method based on CNN for histopathology image analysis on whole slide images. They applied the adaptive sampling technique to overcome issues on larger sizes of images.

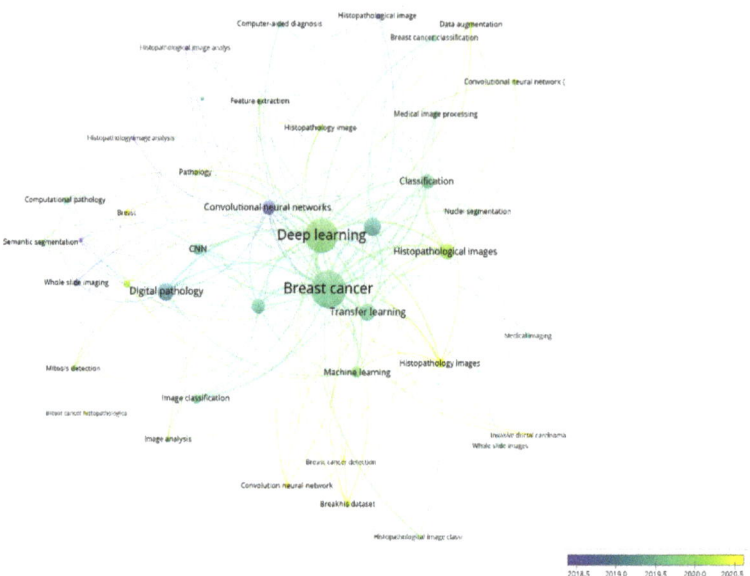

Figure 7. Co-occurrence overlay visualization of keywords in publication for 2014–2021.

Spanhol [12] said that a well-described image database is important for CAD system research, and a new histopathology image dataset known as BreakHis is introduced together with some experimental results using CNN models. Meanwhile, in 2019, Ghosh et al. [88] studied on deep learning and image segmentation and revealed that the medical imaging field needs various segmentations such as nuclei segmentation for reliable CNN performance. Alom et al. [63] proposed an Inception Recurrent Residual Convolutional Neural Network (IRRCNN) model based on several criteria such as magnification factors, image resizing, and image augmentation and segmentation. Result showed that the IRCNN model outperformed the state-of-the art method in 2016 using BreakHis dataset. In 2020, Salama et al. [105] introduced a hybrid deep learning method for breast cancer detection using pre-trained models, ResNet50 and VGG16. Theoretically, a promising accuracy rate depends on the amount of data for model training such that a large volume of training samples leads to a better accuracy rate. Since medical images have a limitation on the sample size, she addressed the limitation by utilizing a data augmentation technique and transfer learning which revealed that hand-crafted features and human interface can be discarded. A hybrid ResNet15 model achieved the highest accuracy, 97.98%, as compared to hybrid VGG16 and other models. However, for this deep learning algorithm to be fully established and exploited on a worldwide scale, significant challenges must be overcome. Some discussion on the challenges of deep learning for breast cancer classification using histopathology images is provided in the next section.

4.7. Computational Method for Histopathology Images

In recent years, there has been a growth and development in the use of deep learning algorithms for histopathology image analysis, specifically CNN methods. CNN methods could be used for identifying regions of interest (ROIs), feature extraction, and image classification. The advent of digital histopathology images with CNN methods offers tremendous potential for assisting pathologists with their jobs. Thereby, Table 7 shows a summary of some deep learning algorithms based on CNN methods in histopathology images. The five listed references are from a high-impact journal with over 100 citations.

Table 7. Five references in publication in high impact journal on CNN methods.

References	Journal	Model/Method	IF [1]	H-Index	Cit [2]	Year
Cruz-Roa et al. [106]	Scientific Reports	CNN/ConvNet	4.380	213	292	2017
Wang H. et al. [51]	Journal of Medical Imaging	CNN and handcrafted features	3.610	29	272	2014
Han Z. et al. [24]	Scientific Reports	Structured based deep CNN	4.380	213	210	2017
Ghosh S. et al. [88]	ACM Computing Surveys	Deep learning, CNN	10.282	163	126	2019
Alom M. Z. et al. [63]	Journal of Digital Imaging	Deep CNN, Inception-v4, ResNet, Recurrent CNN	4.056	58	123	2019

[1] Impact factor; [2] citations.

Cruz-Roa et al. [106] aimed to assess the accuracy and reliability of deep learning algorithms for classifying the digital images into invasive tumor. They offered a novel method for classifying the invasive tumor on whole-slide images using a CNN-based method. In this study, classification performance was assessed across all the images retrieved from the Cancer Institute of New Jersey (CINJ) in the form of whole-slide images. They used three different convolutional network (ConvNet) layers—three-layer ConvNet, four-layer ConvNet, and six-layer ConvNet—as the classifier and compared them with handcrafted features (color, shape, texture, and topography). They concluded that the classification performance related with those features are lower and resulted in higher inconsistency as compared to the ConvNet classifier. Meanwhile, in mitosis detection analysis, the use of handcrafted features solely may result in low accuracy model, whereas CNN methods have issue on high computational cost. Hence, motivated from these drawbacks of handcrafted features and CNN methods, Wang H. et al. [51] introduced a hybrid approach for mitosis detection on ICPR12 dataset. To address these issues, handcrafted features and a CNN method are combined through cascaded ensemble. The results demonstrate that the accuracy of the provided approach still needs to be improved, and a GPU should be used to create a deep multilayer CNN model. Han Z. et al. [24] presented a breast cancer multi-classification technique that makes use of a deep learning model. They implemented a complete recognition approach based on a newly developed class-structure-based deep convolutional neural network (CSDCNN) to provide a consistent and accurate solution for breast cancer classification. They also utilized multi-scale data augmentation and over-sampling approaches to overcome overfitting and unbalanced classes issues. On a large dataset, the proposed CNN model performed admirably.

In Ghosh S. et al. [88], they stated CNN as among the most widely used methods in computer vision. For the segmentation tasks, CNN methods have undergone many basic adjustments to perform effectively. In addition, back-propagation enabled CNN to train a cascaded set of convolutional kernels. It has been greatly improved since then. Generally, they stated that the speed and accuracy of models are important factors in performance evaluation. The speed may be increased through network compression by using depth-wise separable convolutions, kernel factorizations, and a smaller number of spatial convolutions approaches. The popularity of generative adversarial networks (GANs) has recently risen, but there is still some room for improvement in image segmentation. A study by Alom M. Z. et al. [63] demonstrated how deep learning has outperformed state-of-the-art approaches in medical imaging areas. They developed an approach for breast cancer classification known as Inception Recurrent Residual Convolutional Neural Network (IRRCNN) model. This sophisticated DCNN model combines the strengths of the Inception-v4, ResNet, and recurrent CNN (RCNN) with several criteria on data augmentation techniques. Compared with other relevant deep learning algorithms such as inception, RCNN, and residual network, the IRRCNN model offers better performance while utilizing the same or less network parameters.

4.8. Challenges and Future Directions

In this bibliometric analysis, we discovered that deep learning algorithms can be utilized to classify breast cancer histopathology images, given that the model performance (in terms of accuracy) is equal or better as compared to healthcare professionals. However, some parameters must still be considered for a reliable and consistent output. With so much focus on the advancement of deep learning, more individuals are interested in its performance in healthcare.

4.8.1. Large Image Size

In deep learning, image classification frequently utilized small-sized images as an input for the network. Large images have to be resized to fit the network requirement given that a larger size of images leads to a large amount of parameter estimation, computational power, and memory usage. In analysis, whole slide images (WSI) are commonly difficult to be examined, but resizing the images could reduce the information of the cell which leads to less accurate image classification. Therefore, the WSI is often divided into patches (small regions) so that each patch can be evaluated independently. Recently, the findings from Zhou L. et al. [107] demonstrate the benefits of using CNN methods to classify the breast images patch by patch, and the assessment of breast imaging information may yield more accurate and reproducible imaging diagnoses than human interpretation.

4.8.2. Color Variations

For comparable results during analysis, color variation is another issue in deep learning models. Different batches or manufacturers of staining solutions, thickness of tissue sections, staining settings, and scanner models are all sources of variance [49]. Learning without taking color variation into account may degrade the performance of deep learning models. Several techniques have been proposed to deal with the color variation of the images such as color augmentation, color normalization, and grayscale conversion [49]. Grayscale conversion is the simplest method [59], but it may be overlooking critical information on the color representation commonly used by pathologists. Color normalization attempts to change the color values of an image pixel by pixel, using some methods such as color constancy, color deconvolution, and color transfer. Color normalization could be appropriate when the images have identical cell or tissue compositions. However, the utilization of color normalization should be handled carefully because it may reduce the accuracy of the classification algorithm related to histopathology images [108].

4.8.3. Insufficient Data

When there is insufficient data, usually CNN models are less generalized and may lead to an overfitting problem. One approach to avoid the issue is through data augmentation tasks which helps to increase the performance of CNN models in image classification. Recently, automatic approaches to data augmentation, such as data augmentation based on multi degree-of-freedom (DOF) automatic image acquisition, have been presented by Chen L. et al. [109]. It is necessary to assess the physical validity of the created samples and the implications of the several generated problems on the algorithm performance. Several methods for generating synthetic samples using generative adversarial networks have recently been proposed Zhou F. et al. [110]. The generative adversarial network can generate samples in data augmentation tasks rapidly, especially in image-to-image translation [20].

5. Conclusions

The bibliometric analysis study highlights the growing trend of breast cancer and deep learning research globally. This study conducted a bibliometric analysis and visualization of breast cancer image classification using deep learning publications from 2014 to 2021. This study examined some noteworthy findings connected to the related publications. The topic of breast cancer image classification using deep learning has seen a lot of research over the last eight years, with the publications output growing at an exponential rate since 2014. There is a growing interest in breast cancer and deep learning research, which is in response to the pressing demand for urban growth and quality of life. With the technological advancements that have occurred in the last two decades, tremendous progress has been noticed in breast cancer and deep learning studies across all disciplines [93,105].

The main study areas in the realm of breast cancer image classification using deep learning could be recognized based on co-keyword network analysis: (i) breast cancer; (ii) deep learning; (iii) convolutional neural network; (iv) digital pathology; and (v) transfer learning. The theme of the study changed swiftly as time went on, and several fields of breast cancer image classification using deep learning research were thriving at the same time, according to keyword bursts analysis. The histopathology images, invasive ductal carcinoma, and BreakHis dataset have all become new research centers. About 98.54% of authors ($n = 1291/1310$) were credited in not more than three papers on the issue of breast cancer image classification using deep learning, according to co-authorship analyses. This could indicate that a substantial percentage of authors were new to the field of research. Author collaboration network analysis revealed that Li Y., Madabhushi A., and Gilmore H. were among the most productive authors, the most linked authors, and the most cited authors. This suggests that those authors are pioneers in the field of research. Over the past eight years, deep-learning-related methods, especially CNN, have showed outstanding performance in breast cancer image classification. However, data related to medical images or microscopy images are normally limited due to a small number of patients. A large amount of data is required for training the model effectively. Therefore, some researchers used image segmentation techniques to overcome the problem. Data augmentation can help to increase the number of input images by adding copied images from the original input. The new images are slightly modified using several data augmentation strategies such as rotation, flipping, and scaling.

In this study, some challenges related to the CNN method are discussed, and data insufficiency might be the biggest challenge in medical data for image classification. This is also supported by Komura and Ishikawa [49]: their work stated that a large amount of training data is important for image classification tasks. A vast amount of research has been conducted on CNN methods with several adjustment to reach model efficiency of image classification specifically on breast cancer histopathology images. As discussed in the previous section, recently, some studies revealed that generative adversarial networks (GANs) could be used to generate samples for training datasets, so that issue on data scarcity can be tackled. The implementation of GANs in future studies as a data synthesis option should be further explored to elevate the computational time and improve the performance of the CNN methods.

VOSviewer used country collaboration analysis to divide the 35 countries into nine research strong-linked clusters, led by the United States, China, India, South Korea, and the United Kingdom, respectively. They were also at the forefront of a collaborative effort to classify breast cancer images using deep learning. The United States and China were both ranked in the top two in author collaboration and country collaboration analyses. China, on the other hand, has recently adopted a more cooperative attitude. In fact, China is one of the world's newest scientific hubs.

This bibliometric study has some limitations to be addressed. First, the data collection was restricted to Scopus' core collection, with improvements such as "source type" and "languages" being used. Other databases such as PubMed or WoS should have been combined as well. Nonetheless, Scopus is one of the world's largest and most utilized databases for scientific publication analysis, particularly in the healthcare area. Second, since some recently published papers have low citation frequency, there may still be discrepancies between true research status and our bibliometric analysis results [111]. As a conclusion, the role of deep learning in breast cancer image classification will keep evolving. However, deep learning is not a replacement for pathologists; instead, it will continue to assist them with tools that are both effective and efficient. This bibliometric analysis could be used as a springboard for more specific and in-depth research.

Author Contributions: Conceptualization, S.S.M.K. and C.-Y.L.; methodology, S.S.M.K.; software, S.S.M.K.; resources, C.-Y.L.; writing—original draft preparation, S.S.M.K.; writing—review and editing, C.-Y.L., M.A.A., M.A.A.B., S.A.B., N.R. and M.F.; visualization, S.S.M.K.; supervision, C.-Y.L., M.A.A., M.A.A.B., S.A.B., N.R. and M.F. All authors have read and agreed to the published version of the manuscript.

Funding: This research is funded by the National University of Malaysia (UKM) with the grant number is DIP-2018-039.

Institutional Review Board Statement: Not applicable.

Informed Consent Statement: Not applicable.

Data Availability Statement: The data presented in this study are available on request from the corresponding author.

Acknowledgments: It is with the deepest regret that we record the death of Choong-Yeun Liong on 25 September 2021. His contributions as main person in supervision will be sorely missed. He was a well-loved colleague at the National University of Malaysia (UKM) for many years.

Conflicts of Interest: The authors declare no conflict of interest.

References

1. Nenclares, P.; Harrington, K.J. The Biology of Cancer. *Medicine* **2020**, *48*, 67–72. [CrossRef]
2. Bray, F.; Ferlay, J.; Soerjomataram, I.; Siegel, R.L.; Torre, L.A.; Jemal, A. Global Cancer Statistics 2018: GLOBOCAN Estimates of Incidence and Mortality Worldwide for 36 Cancers in 185 Countries. *CA Cancer J. Clin.* **2018**, *68*, 394–424. [CrossRef]
3. Siegel, R.L.; Miller, K.D.; Jemal, A. Cancer Statistics, 2020. *CA Cancer J. Clin.* **2020**, *70*, 7–30. [CrossRef] [PubMed]
4. Torre, L.A.; Siegel, R.L.; Ward, E.M.; Jemal, A. Global Cancer Incidence and Mortality Rates and Trends—An Update. *Cancer Epidemiol. Biomark. Prev.* **2016**, *25*, 16–27. [CrossRef]
5. Sung, H.; Ferlay, J.; Siegel, R.L.; Laversanne, M.; Soerjomataram, I.; Jemal, A.; Bray, F. Global Cancer Statistics 2020: GLOBOCAN Estimates of Incidence and Mortality Worldwide for 36 Cancers in 185 Countries. *CA Cancer J. Clin.* **2021**, *71*, 209–249. [CrossRef]
6. Momenimovahed, Z.; Salehiniya, H. Epidemiological Characteristics of and Risk Factors for Breast Cancer in the World. *Breast Cancer Targets Ther.* **2019**, *11*, 151–164. [CrossRef] [PubMed]
7. Abdelwahab Yousef, A.J. Male Breast Cancer: Epidemiology and Risk Factors. *Semin. Oncol.* **2017**, *44*, 267–272. [CrossRef] [PubMed]
8. Nahid, A.-A.; Kong, Y. Involvement of Machine Learning for Breast Cancer Image Classification: A Survey. *Comput. Math. Methods Med.* **2017**, *2017*, 3781951. [CrossRef] [PubMed]
9. Skandalakis, J.E. Embryology and Anatomy of the Breast. In *Breast Augmentation*; Shiffman, M., Ed.; Springer: Berlin/Heidelberg, Germany, 2009; pp. 3–24. ISBN 978-3-540-78948-2.
10. Bombonati, A.; Sgroi, D.C. The Molecular Pathology of Breast Cancer Progression. *J. Pathol.* **2011**, *223*, 308–318. [CrossRef]
11. Gajdosova, V.; Lorencova, L.; Kasak, P.; Tkac, J. Electrochemical Nanobiosensors for Detection of Breast Cancer Biomarkers. *Sensors* **2020**, *20*, 4022. [CrossRef] [PubMed]
12. Spanhol, F.A. Automatic Breast Cancer Classification from Histopathological Images: A Hybrid Approach. Ph.D. Thesis, Federal University of Parana, Curitiba, Brazil, 2018.
13. Liu, Y.; Ren, L.; Cao, X.; Tong, Y. Breast Tumors Recognition Based on Edge Feature Extraction Using Support Vector Machine. *Biomed. Signal Process. Control* **2020**, *58*, 101825. [CrossRef]
14. Danch-Wierzchowska, M.; Borys, D.; Bobek-Bilewicz, B.; Jarzab, M.; Swierniak, A. Simplification of Breast Deformation Modelling to Support Breast Cancer Treatment Planning. *Biocybern. Biomed. Eng.* **2016**, *36*, 531–536. [CrossRef]
15. Mewada, H.K.; Patel, A.V.; Hassaballah, M.; Alkinani, M.H.; Mahant, K. Spectral–Spatial Features Integrated Convolution Neural Network for Breast Cancer Classification. *Sensors* **2020**, *20*, 4747. [CrossRef] [PubMed]
16. Kiambe, K.; Kiambe, K. Breast Histopathological Image Feature Extraction with Convolutional Neural Networks for Classification. *ICSES Trans. Image Process. Pattern Recognit. (ITIPPR)* **2018**, *4*, 4–12. [CrossRef]
17. Mathew, T.; Kini, J.R.; Rajan, J. Computational Methods for Automated Mitosis Detection in Histopathology Images: A Review. *Biocybern. Biomed. Eng.* **2021**, *41*, 64–82. [CrossRef]
18. Zhu, C.; Song, F.; Wang, Y.; Dong, H.; Guo, Y.; Liu, J. Breast Cancer Histopathology Image Classification through Assembling Multiple Compact CNNs. *BMC Med. Inform. Decis. Mak.* **2019**, *19*, 198. [CrossRef] [PubMed]

19. Valieris, R.; Amaro, L.; de Toledo Osório, C.A.B.; Bueno, A.P.; Mitrowsky, R.A.R.; Carraro, D.M.; Nunes, D.N.; Dias-Neto, E.; da Silva, I.T. Deep Learning Predicts Underlying Features on Pathology Images with Therapeutic Relevance for Breast and Gastric Cancer. *Cancers* **2020**, *12*, 3687. [CrossRef]
20. Lagree, A.; Mohebpour, M.; Meti, N.; Saednia, K.; Lu, F.I.; Slodkowska, E.; Gandhi, S.; Rakovitch, E.; Shenfield, A.; Sadeghi-Naini, A.; et al. A Review and Comparison of Breast Tumor Cell Nuclei Segmentation Performances Using Deep Convolutional Neural Networks. *Sci. Rep.* **2021**, *11*, 8025. [CrossRef]
21. Choudhary, T.; Mishra, V.; Goswami, A.; Sarangapani, J. A Transfer Learning with Structured Filter Pruning Approach for Improved Breast Cancer Classification on Point-of-Care Devices. *Comput. Biol. Med.* **2021**, *134*, 104432. [CrossRef]
22. Kozegar, E.; Soryani, M.; Behnam, H.; Salamati, M.; Tan, T. Computer Aided Detection in Automated 3-D Breast Ultrasound Images: A Survey. *Artif. Intell. Rev.* **2020**, *53*, 1919–1941. [CrossRef]
23. Murtaza, G.; Shuib, L.; Abdul Wahab, A.W.; Mujtaba, G.; Mujtaba, G.; Nweke, H.F.; Al-garadi, M.A.; Zulfiqar, F.; Raza, G.; Azmi, N.A. Deep Learning-Based Breast Cancer Classification through Medical Imaging Modalities: State of the Art and Research Challenges. *Artif. Intell. Rev.* **2020**, *53*, 1655–1720. [CrossRef]
24. Han, Z.; Wei, B.; Zheng, Y.; Yin, Y.; Li, K.; Li, S. Breast Cancer Multi-Classification from Histopathological Images with Structured Deep Learning Model. *Sci. Rep.* **2017**, *7*, 4172. [CrossRef] [PubMed]
25. Rezaeilouyeh, H.; Mollahosseini, A.; Mahoor, M.H. Microscopic Medical Image Classification Framework via Deep Learning and Shearlet Transform. *J. Med. Imaging* **2016**, *3*, 044501. [CrossRef]
26. Pizarro, R.A.; Cheng, X.; Barnett, A.; Lemaitre, H.; Verchinski, B.A.; Goldman, A.L.; Xiao, E.; Luo, Q.; Berman, K.F.; Callicott, J.H.; et al. Automated Quality Assessment of Structural Magnetic Resonance Brain Images Based on a Supervised Machine Learning Algorithm. *Front. Neuroinform.* **2016**, *10*, 52. [CrossRef]
27. Farjam, R.; Soltanian-Zadeh, H.; Zoroofi, R.A.; Jafari-Khouzani, K. Tree-Structured Grading of Pathological Images of Prostate. In Proceedings of the SPIE 5747, Medical Imaging 2005: Image Processing, San Diego, CA, USA, 29 April 2005; pp. 1–12. [CrossRef]
28. Wang, P.; Hu, X.; Li, Y.; Liu, Q.; Zhu, X. Automatic Cell Nuclei Segmentation and Classification of Breast Cancer Histopathology Images. *Signal Process.* **2016**, *122*, 1–13. [CrossRef]
29. Lopez Martinez, R.E.; Sierra, G. Research Trends in the International Literature on Natural Language Processing, 2000–2019—A Bibliometric Study. *J. Scientometr. Res.* **2020**, *9*, 310–318. [CrossRef]
30. Ahmi, A.; Mohamad, R. Bibliometric Analysis of Global Scientific Literature on Web Accessibility. *Int. J. Recent Technol. Eng.* **2019**, *7*, 250–258.
31. Marczewska, M.; Kostrzewski, M. Sustainable Business Models: A Bibliometric Performance Analysis. *Energies* **2020**, *13*, 6062. [CrossRef]
32. de las Heras-Rosas, C.; Herrera, J.; Rodríguez-Fernández, M. Organisational Commitment in Healthcare Systems: A Bibliometric Analysis. *Int. J. Environ. Res. Public Health* **2021**, *18*, 2271. [CrossRef]
33. Ozen Çınar, İ. Bibliometric Analysis of Breast Cancer Research in the Period 2009–2018. *Int. J. Nurs. Pract.* **2020**, *26*, e12845. [CrossRef] [PubMed]
34. Salod, Z.; Singh, Y. A Five-Year (2015 to 2019) Analysis of Studies Focused on Breast Cancer Prediction Using Machine Learning: A Systematic Review and Bibliometric Analysis. *J. Public Health Res.* **2020**, *9*, 65–75. [CrossRef]
35. Joshi, S.A.; Bongale, A.M.; Bongale, A. Breast Cancer Detection from Histopathology Images Using Machine Learning Techniques: A Bibliometric Analysis. *Libr. Philos. Pract.* **2021**, *5376*, 1–29.
36. Erickson, B.J.; Korfiatis, P.; Akkus, Z.; Kline, T.L. Machine Learning for Medical Imaging. *Radiographics* **2017**, *37*, 505–515. [CrossRef]
37. Bengio, Y. Learning Deep Architectures for AI. In *Foundations and Trends®in Machine Learning*; University of California: Berkeley, CA, USA, 2009; Volume 2, pp. 1–127. [CrossRef]
38. Li, X.; Shen, X.; Zhou, Y.; Wang, X.; Li, T.-Q. Classification of Breast Cancer Histopathological Images Using Interleaved DenseNet with SENet (IDSNet). *PLoS ONE* **2020**, *15*, e0232127. [CrossRef] [PubMed]
39. Spanhol, F.A.; Oliveira, L.S.; Petitjean, C.; Heutte, L. A Dataset for Breast Cancer Histopathological Image Classification. *IEEE Trans. Biomed. Eng.* **2016**, *63*, 1455–1462. [CrossRef]
40. Aresta, G.; Araújo, T.; Kwok, S.; Chennamsetty, S.S.; Safwan, M.; Alex, V.; Marami, B.; Prastawa, M.; Chan, M.; Donovan, M.; et al. BACH: Grand Challenge on Breast Cancer Histology Images. *Med. Image Anal.* **2019**, *56*, 122–139. [CrossRef]
41. Asri, H.; Mousannif, H.; Moatassime, H.A.; Noel, T. Using Machine Learning Algorithms for Breast Cancer Risk Prediction and Diagnosis. *Procedia Comput. Sci.* **2016**, *83*, 1064–1069. [CrossRef]
42. Bharat, A.; Pooja, N.; Reddy, R.A. Using Machine Learning Algorithms for Breast Cancer Risk Prediction and Diagnosis. In Proceedings of the 2018 3rd International Conference on Circuits, Control, Communication and Computing (I4C), Bangalore, India, 3–5 October 2018; pp. 1–4. [CrossRef]
43. Zhang, Y.; Deng, Q.; Liang, W.; Zou, X. An Efficient Feature Selection Strategy Based on Multiple Support Vector Machine Technology with Gene Expression Data. *Biomed Res. Int.* **2018**, *2018*, 7538204. [CrossRef] [PubMed]
44. Kharya, S.; Agrawal, S.; Soni, S. Naive Bayes Classifiers: A Probabilistic Detection Model for Breast Cancer. *Int. J. Comput. Appl.* **2014**, *92*, 26–31. [CrossRef]
45. Nahar, J.; Chen, Y.P.P.; Ali, S. Kernel-Based Naive Bayes Classifier for Breast Cancer Prediction. *J. Biol. Syst.* **2007**, *15*, 17–25. [CrossRef]

46. Rashmi, G.D.; Lekha, A.; Bawane, N. Analysis of Efficiency of Classification and Prediction Algorithms (Naïve Bayes) for Breast Cancer Dataset. In Proceedings of the 2015 International Conference on Emerging Research in Electronics, Computer Science and Technology (ICERECT), Mandya, India, 17–19 December 2015; pp. 108–113.
47. Octaviani, T.L.; Rustam, Z. Random Forest for Breast Cancer Prediction. In Proceedings of the AIP Conference Proceedings, Depok, Indonesia, 30–31 October 2018; pp. 1–7. [CrossRef]
48. Elgedawy, M.N. Prediction of Breast Cancer Using Random Forest, Support Vector Machines and Naïve Bayes. *Int. J. Eng. Comput. Sci.* **2017**, *6*, 19884–19889. [CrossRef]
49. Komura, D.; Ishikawa, S. Machine Learning Methods for Histopathological Image Analysis. *Comput. Struct. Biotechnol. J.* **2018**, *16*, 34–42. [CrossRef] [PubMed]
50. LeCun, Y.; Bengio, Y.; Hinton, G. Deep Learning. *Nature* **2015**, *521*, 436–444. [CrossRef]
51. Wang, H.; Cruz-Roa, A.; Basavanhally, A.; Gilmore, H.; Shih, N.; Feldman, M.; Tomaszewski, J.; Gonzalez, F.; Madabhushi, A. Mitosis Detection in Breast Cancer Pathology Images by Combining Handcrafted and Convolutional Neural Network Features. *J. Med. Imaging* **2014**, *1*, 034003. [CrossRef] [PubMed]
52. Shahidi, F.; Daud, S.M.; Abas, H.; Ahmad, N.A.; Maarop, N. Breast Cancer Classification Using Deep Learning Approaches and Histopathology Image: A Comparison Study. *IEEE Access* **2020**, *8*, 187531–187552. [CrossRef]
53. Fujita, H. AI-Based Computer-Aided Diagnosis (AI-CAD): The Latest Review to Read First. *Radiol. Phys. Technol.* **2020**, *13*, 6–19. [CrossRef]
54. Lin, C.J.; Jeng, S.Y. Optimization of Deep Learning Network Parameters Using Uniform Experimental Design for Breast Cancer Histopathological Image Classification. *Diagnostics* **2020**, *10*, 662. [CrossRef] [PubMed]
55. Schmidhuber, J. Deep Learning in Neural Networks: An Overview. *Neural Netw.* **2015**, *61*, 85–117. [CrossRef]
56. Mishra, C.; Gupta, D.L. Deep Machine Learning and Neural Networks: An Overview. *IAES Int. J. Artif. Intell.* **2017**, *6*, 66–73. [CrossRef]
57. Nguyen, P.T.; Nguyen, T.T.; Nguyen, N.C.; Le, T.T. Multiclass Breast Cancer Classification Using Convolutional Neural Network. In Proceedings of the 2019 International Symposium on Electrical and Electronics Engineering (ISEE), Ho Chi Minh City, Vietnam, 10–12 October 2019; pp. 130–134. [CrossRef]
58. Bengio, Y.; Lee, H. Editorial Introduction to the Neural Networks Special Issue on Deep Learning of Representations. *Neural Netw.* **2015**, *64*, 1–3. [CrossRef]
59. Hirra, I.; Ahmad, M.; Hussain, A.; Ashraf, M.U.; Saeed, I.A.; Qadri, S.F.; Alghamdi, A.M.; Alfakeeh, A.S. Breast Cancer Classification from Histopathological Images Using Patch-Based Deep Learning Modeling. *IEEE Access* **2021**, *9*, 24273–24287. [CrossRef]
60. Zuluaga-Gomez, J.; Al Masry, Z.; Benaggoune, K.; Meraghni, S.; Zerhouni, N. A CNN-Based Methodology for Breast Cancer Diagnosis Using Thermal Images. *Comput. Methods Biomech. Biomed. Eng. Imaging Vis.* **2021**, *9*, 131–145. [CrossRef]
61. Hameed, Z.; Zahia, S.; Garcia-Zapirain, B.; Aguirre, J.J.; Vanegas, A.M. Breast Cancer Histopathology Image Classification Using an Ensemble of Deep Learning Models. *Sensors* **2020**, *20*, 4373. [CrossRef] [PubMed]
62. Pavithra, P.; Ravichandran, K.S.; Sekar, K.R.; Manikandan, R. The Effect of Thermography on Breast Cancer Detection—A Survey. *Syst. Rev. Pharm.* **2018**, *9*, 10–16. [CrossRef]
63. Alom, M.Z.; Yakopcic, C.; Nasrin, M.S.; Taha, T.M.; Asari, V.K. Breast Cancer Classification from Histopathological Images with Inception Recurrent Residual Convolutional Neural Network. *J. Digit. Imaging* **2019**, *32*, 605–617. [CrossRef] [PubMed]
64. Železnik, D.; Blažun Vošner, H.; Kokol, P. A Bibliometric Analysis of the Journal of Advanced Nursing, 1976–2015. *J. Adv. Nurs.* **2017**, *73*, 2407–2419. [CrossRef] [PubMed]
65. Liao, H.; Tang, M.; Luo, L.; Li, C.; Chiclana, F.; Zeng, X.J. A Bibliometric Analysis and Visualization of Medical Big Data Research. *Sustainability* **2018**, *10*, 166. [CrossRef]
66. Guo, Y.; Hao, Z.; Zhao, S.; Gong, J.; Yang, F. Artificial Intelligence in Health Care: Bibliometric Analysis. *J. Med. Internet Res.* **2020**, *22*, e18228. [CrossRef]
67. Bhattacharya, S. Some Salient Aspects of Machine Learning Research: A Bibliometric Analysis. *J. Scientometr. Res.* **2019**, *8*, 85–92. [CrossRef]
68. Aria, M.; Cuccurullo, C. Bibliometrix: An R-Tool for Comprehensive Science Mapping Analysis. *J. Informetr.* **2017**, *11*, 959–975. [CrossRef]
69. van Eck, N.J.; Waltman, L. Software Survey: VOSviewer, a Computer Program for Bibliometric Mapping. *Scientometrics* **2010**, *84*, 523–538. [CrossRef]
70. Wahid, R.; Ahmi, A.; Alam, A.S.A.F. Growth and Collaboration in Massive Open Online Courses: A Bibliometric Analysis. *Int. Rev. Res. Open Distance Learn.* **2020**, *21*, 292–322. [CrossRef]
71. Baas, J.; Schotten, M.; Plume, A.; Côté, G.; Karimi, R. Scopus as a Curated, High-Quality Bibliometric Data Source for Academic Research in Quantitative Science Studies. *Quant. Sci. Stud.* **2020**, *1*, 377–386. [CrossRef]
72. Tober, M. PubMed, ScienceDirect, Scopus or Google Scholar—Which Is the Best Search Engine for an Effective Literature Research in Laser Medicine? *Med. Laser Appl.* **2011**, *26*, 139–144. [CrossRef]
73. Al-antari, M.A.; Han, S.-M.; Kim, T.-S. Evaluation of Deep Learning Detection and Classification towards Computer-Aided Diagnosis of Breast Lesions in Digital X-Ray Mammograms. *Comput. Methods Programs Biomed.* **2020**, *196*, 105584. [CrossRef] [PubMed]

74. Swiderski, B.; Kurek, J.; Osowski, S.; Kruk, M.; Barhoumi, W. Deep Learning and Non-Negative Matrix Factorization in Recognition of Mammograms. In Proceedings of the Eighth International Conference on Graphic and Image Processing (ICGIP 2016), Tokyo, Japan, 29–31 October 2016; pp. 1–7. [CrossRef]
75. Grover, S.; Dalton, N. Abstract to Publication Rate: Do All the Papers Presented in Conferences See the Light of Being a Full Publication? *Indian J. Psychiatry* **2020**, *62*, 73–79. [CrossRef] [PubMed]
76. Bar-Ilan, J. Web of Science with the Conference Proceedings Citation Indexes: The Case of Computer Science. *Scientometrics* **2010**, *83*, 809–824. [CrossRef]
77. Purnell, P.J. Conference Proceedings Publications in Bibliographic Databases: A Case Study of Countries in Southeast Asia. *Scientometrics* **2021**, *126*, 355–387. [CrossRef]
78. Janowczyk, A.; Madabhushi, A. Deep Learning for Digital Pathology Image Analysis: A Comprehensive Tutorial with Selected Use Cases. *J. Pathol. Inform.* **2016**, *7*, 29. [CrossRef] [PubMed]
79. Nagpal, K.; Foote, D.; Liu, Y.; Chen, P.H.C.; Wulczyn, E.; Tan, F.; Olson, N.; Smith, J.L.; Mohtashamian, A.; Wren, J.H.; et al. Development and Validation of a Deep Learning Algorithm for Improving Gleason Scoring of Prostate Cancer. *NPJ Digit. Med.* **2019**, *2*, 48. [CrossRef]
80. Bejnordi, B.E.; Veta, M.; Van Diest, P.J.; Van Ginneken, B.; Karssemeijer, N.; Litjens, G.; Van Der Laak, J.A.W.M.; Hermsen, M.; Manson, Q.F.; Balkenhol, M.; et al. Diagnostic Assessment of Deep Learning Algorithms for Detection of Lymph Node Metastases in Women with Breast Cancer. *JAMA J. Am. Med. Assoc.* **2017**, *318*, 2199–2210. [CrossRef] [PubMed]
81. Bera, K.; Schalper, K.A.; Rimm, D.L.; Velcheti, V.; Madabhushi, A. Diagnosis and Precision Oncology. *Nat. Rev. Clin. Oncol.* **2019**, *16*, 703–715. [CrossRef]
82. Zakaria, R.; Ahmi, A.; Ahmad, A.H.; Othman, Z.; Azman, K.F.; Ab Aziz, C.B.; Ismail, C.A.N.; Shafin, N. Visualising and Mapping a Decade of Literature on Honey Research: A Bibliometric Analysis from 2011 to 2020. *J. Apic. Res.* **2021**, *60*, 359–368. [CrossRef]
83. Bongaarts, J. United Nations Department of Economic and Social Affairs, Population DivisionWorld Family Planning 2020: Highlights, United Nations Publications, 2020. 46 P. *Popul. Dev. Rev.* **2020**, *46*, 857–858. [CrossRef]
84. Peters, H.P.F.; van Raan, A.F.J. Co-Word-Based Science Maps of Chemical Engineering. Part II: Representations by Combined Clustering and Multidimensional Scaling. *Res. Policy* **1993**, *22*, 47–71. [CrossRef]
85. Waltman, L.; van Eck, N.J.; Noyons, E.C.M. A Unified Approach to Mapping and Clustering of Bibliometric Networks. *J. Informetr.* **2010**, *4*, 629–635. [CrossRef]
86. Kumar, A.; Singh, S.K.; Saxena, S.; Lakshmanan, K.; Sangaiah, A.K.; Chauhan, H.; Shrivastava, S.; Singh, R.K. Deep Feature Learning for Histopathological Image Classification of Canine Mammary Tumors and Human Breast Cancer. *Inf. Sci.* **2020**, *508*, 405–421. [CrossRef]
87. Zhang, Y.D.; Satapathy, S.C.; Guttery, D.S.; Górriz, J.M.; Wang, S.H. Improved Breast Cancer Classification Through Combining Graph Convolutional Network and Convolutional Neural Network. *Inf. Process. Manag.* **2021**, *58*, 102439. [CrossRef]
88. Ghosh, S.; Das, N.; Das, I.; Maulik, U. Understanding Deep Learning Techniques for Image Segmentation. *ACM Comput. Surv.* **2019**, *52*, 1–35. [CrossRef]
89. Sudharshan, P.J.; Petitjean, C.; Spanhol, F.; Oliveira, L.E.; Heutte, L.; Honeine, P. Multiple Instance Learning for Histopathological Breast Cancer Image Classification. *Expert Syst. Appl.* **2019**, *117*, 103–111. [CrossRef]
90. Xu, J.; Xiang, L.; Liu, Q.; Gilmore, H.; Wu, J.; Tang, J.; Madabhushi, A. Stacked Sparse Autoencoder (SSAE) for Nuclei Detection on Breast Cancer Histopathology Images. *IEEE Trans. Med. Imaging* **2016**, *35*, 119–130. [CrossRef] [PubMed]
91. Chen, H.; Deng, Z. Bibliometric Analysis of the Application of Convolutional Neural Network in Computer Vision. *IEEE Access* **2020**, *8*, 155417–155428. [CrossRef]
92. e Fonseca, B.D.P.F.; Sampaio, R.B.; de Fonseca, M.V.; Zicker, F. Co-Authorship Network Analysis in Health Research: Method and Potential Use. *Health Res. Policy Syst.* **2016**, *14*, 34. [CrossRef]
93. Wang, P.; Wang, J.; Li, Y.; Li, P.; Li, L.; Jiang, M. Automatic Classification of Breast Cancer Histopathological Images Based on Deep Feature Fusion and Enhanced Routing. *Biomed. Signal Process. Control* **2021**, *65*, 102341. [CrossRef]
94. Elmannai, H.; Hamdi, M.; AlGarni, A. Deep Learning Models Combining for Breast Cancer Histopathology Image Classification. *Int. J. Comput. Intell. Syst.* **2021**, *14*, 102341. [CrossRef]
95. Chen, K.; Yao, Q.; Sun, J.; He, Z.; Yao, L.; Liu, Z. International Publication Trends and Collaboration Performance of China in Healthcare Science and Services Research. *Isr. J. Health Policy Res.* **2016**, *5*, 1. [CrossRef] [PubMed]
96. Ahmad, S.; Ur Rehman, S.; Iqbal, A.; Farooq, R.K.; Shahid, A.; Ullah, M.I. Breast Cancer Research in Pakistan: A Bibliometric Analysis. *SAGE Open* **2021**, *11*, 1–17. [CrossRef]
97. Rangarajan, B.; Shet, T.; Wadasadawala, T.; Nair, N.S.; Sairam, R.M.; Hingmire, S.S.; Bajpai, J. Breast Cancer: An Overview of Published Indian Data. *South Asian J. Cancer* **2016**, *5*, 86–92. [CrossRef]
98. Fitzmaurice, C.; Abate, D.; Abbasi, N.; Abbastabar, H.; Abd-Allah, F.; Abdel-Rahman, O.; Abdelalim, A.; Abdoli, A.; Abdollahpour, I.; Abdulle, A.S.M.; et al. Global, Regional, and National Cancer Incidence, Mortality, Years of Life Lost, Years Lived With Disability, and Disability-Adjusted Life-Years for 29 Cancer Groups, 1990 to 2017. *JAMA Oncol.* **2019**, *5*, 1749–1768. [CrossRef]
99. Cruz-Roa, A.; Gilmore, H.; Basavanhally, A.; Feldman, M.; Ganesan, S.; Shih, N.; Tomaszewski, J.; Madabhushi, A.; González, F. High-Throughput Adaptive Sampling for Whole-Slide Histopathology Image Analysis (HASHI) via Convolutional Neural Networks: Application to Invasive Breast Cancer Detection. *PLoS ONE* **2018**, *13*, e0196828. [CrossRef]

100. Lu, C.; Xu, H.; Xu, J.; Gilmore, H.; Mandal, M.; Madabhushi, A. Multi-Pass Adaptive Voting for Nuclei Detection in Histopathological Images. *Sci. Rep.* **2016**, *6*, 33985. [CrossRef]
101. Xu, J.; Xiang, L.; Wang, G.; Ganesan, S.; Feldman, M.; Shih, N.N.; Gilmore, H.; Madabhushi, A. Sparse Non-Negative Matrix Factorization (SNMF) Based Color Unmixing for Breast Histopathological Image Analysis. *Comput. Med. Imaging Graph.* **2015**, *46*, 20–29. [CrossRef] [PubMed]
102. Samb, B.; Desai, N.; Nishtar, S.; Mendis, S.; Bekedam, H.; Wright, A.; Hsu, J.; Martiniuk, A.; Celletti, F.; Patel, K.; et al. Prevention and Management of Chronic Disease: A Litmus Test for Health-Systems Strengthening in Low-Income and Middle-Income Countries. *Lancet* **2010**, *376*, 1785–1797. [CrossRef]
103. Ghosh, P.; Azam, S.; Hasib, K.M.; Karim, A.; Jonkman, M.; Anwar, A. A Performance Based Study on Deep Learning Algorithms in the Effective Prediction of Breast Cancer. In Proceedings of the International Joint Conference on Neural Networks, Shenzhen, China, 18–22 July 2021; pp. 1–8. [CrossRef]
104. Mahmood, T.; Li, J.; Pei, Y.; Akhtar, F.; Jia, Y.; Khand, Z.H. Breast Mass Detection and Classification Using Deep Convolutional Neural Networks for Radiologist Diagnosis Assistance. In Proceedings of the 2021 IEEE 45th Annual Computers, Software, and Applications Conference, COMPSAC 2021, Madrid, Spain, 12–16 July 2021; pp. 1918–1923. [CrossRef]
105. Salama, W.M.; Elbagoury, A.M.; Aly, M.H. Novel Breast Cancer Classification Framework Based on Deep Learning. *IET Image Process.* **2020**, *14*, 3254–3259. [CrossRef]
106. Cruz-Roa, A.; Gilmore, H.; Basavanhally, A.; Feldman, M.; Ganesan, S.; Shih, N.N.C.; Tomaszewski, J.; González, F.A.; Madabhushi, A. Accurate and Reproducible Invasive Breast Cancer Detection in Whole-Slide Images: A Deep Learning Approach for Quantifying Tumor Extent. *Sci. Rep.* **2017**, *7*, 46450. [CrossRef]
107. Zhou, L.; Wei, Q.; Dietrich, C.F. Lymph Node Metastasis Prediction from Primary Breast. *Radiology* **2019**, *294*, 19–24. [CrossRef]
108. Bianconi, F.; Kather, J.N.; Reyes-Aldasoro, C.C. Evaluation of Colour Pre-Processing on Patch-Based Classification of H&E-Stained Images. In *Lecture Notes in Computer Science (Including Subseries Lecture Notes in Artificial Intelligence and Lecture Notes in Bioinformatics)*; Springer: Cham, Switzerland, 2019; pp. 56–64. [CrossRef]
109. Chen, L.; Yan, N.; Yang, H.; Zhu, L.; Zheng, Z.; Yang, X.; Zhang, X. A Data Augmentation Method for Deep Learning Based on Multi-Degree of Freedom (Dof) Automatic Image Acquisition. *Appl. Sci.* **2020**, *10*, 7755. [CrossRef]
110. Zhou, F.; Yang, S.; Fujita, H.; Chen, D.; Wen, C. Deep Learning Fault Diagnosis Method Based on Global Optimization GAN for Unbalanced Data. *Knowl.-Based Syst.* **2020**, *187*, 104837. [CrossRef]
111. Stephan, P.; Veugelers, R.; Wang, J. Reviewers are Blinkered by Bibliometrics. *Nature* **2017**, *544*, 411–412. [CrossRef] [PubMed]

MDPI
St. Alban-Anlage 66
4052 Basel
Switzerland
Tel. +41 61 683 77 34
Fax +41 61 302 89 18
www.mdpi.com

Healthcare Editorial Office
E-mail: healthcare@mdpi.com
www.mdpi.com/journal/healthcare

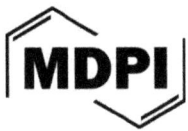